BABY LORE

SUPERSTITIONS & OLD WIVES TALES FROM THE WORLD OVER RELATED TO PREGNANCY, BIRTH & BABYCARE

By Rosalind Franklin

Diggory Press

Copyright 2005

Rosalind Franklin has asserted her right to be identified as the author of this work under the Copyright, Designs & Patents Act 1988

All rights reserved. No parts of this publication may be reproduced, stored in a retrieval system, or transmitted in any form or by any means, electronic, mechanical, photocopying, recording or otherwise without the prior permission of the copyright owner.

Text & Cover Design by Rosalind Franklin

ISBN 0-9515655-4-0

First Published in the United Kingdom, February 2005 by Diggory Press,
an imprint of Meadow Books,
35 Stonefield Way, Burgess Hill, West Sussex, RH15 8DW, UK

Email: Meadowbooks@hotmail.com

INTRODUCTION

When I announced I was pregnant with my first child, I was amazed at what my normally sensible and down-to-earth mother started coming out with.

'Make sure you eat plenty of spinach to make the baby's hair curl,' she said, 'and don't forget to stay out of the sun so Baby doesn't get too hot!' As my mother is a qualified midwife, I expected her to know better. I soon discovered as my pregnancy progressed that midwives are the worst of the lot when it comes to harbouring superstitions about the unborn child.

'The heartbeat's under 140, I'll put money on it that your baby is a boy,' said my own midwife at one of my check-ups (she turned out to be right).

As other female friends and relatives dispensed their own pearls of wisdom about the shape of my ever-expanding belly, I decided to discover just how widespread these 'quaint' superstitions were. I imagined I might find fifty or so baby-related beliefs to giggle at. As I came across literally *thousands* of superstitions, I became amazed at the sheer range and variety of beliefs. Some of these superstitions made me laugh, some made me cry, some made me downright angry. However, all of them held me fascinated, so much so that this book came into being.

I have collected these beliefs from the world over. When I have stated the country where a particular notion is held, I'm not inferring the whole nation adheres to it, neither am I saying that place is the only location where that specific belief is held. It's amazing that despite being miles apart, many countries believe exactly the same thing as each other.

Furthermore, *some* of the superstitions I have listed are now outdated. So for example, the 'fairy changeling' belief, widely accepted as fact up until the beginning of the First World War, now remains only in the memories of our Grandmothers' generation, in the UK at least. However, the less brutal methods of protection against a baby becoming an abducted 'changeling' have stayed in handed-down customs. Many mothers still refuse to dress their newborn in green, although they will not know *why*. The original reason, green being the favoured colour of the fairy baby abductors, has long been forgotten.

Lastly, I have used the phrase 'he' for the baby's gender identity throughout the book for the sake of clarity and consistency. I'm in no way inferring the beliefs relate to only boys, unless I have specifically said so with that particular superstition.

Rosalind Franklin, February 2005

INDEX

PART I	CONCEPTION	
Chapter 1	General Superstitions	9
Chapter 2	Fertility Charms & Amulets	19
Chapter 3	Religious Beliefs	24
Chapter 4	The Powers of Nature	28
Chapter 5	Food & Fertility	41
Chapter 6	The Infant's Sex	44

PART II	PREGNANCY	
Chapter 7	Eating & Drinking	50
Chapter 8	Pregnancy Dangers	55
Chapter 9	Health and Beauty	66
Chapter 10	Other Pregnancy Beliefs	72

PART III	LABOUR & DELIVERY	
Chapter 11	Labour Superstitions	78
Chapter 12	Post Delivery Beliefs	92
Chapter 13	Birth Omens	97
Chapter 14	Timing is Everything	105

PART IV	THE NEWBORN & NEW PARENTS	
Chapter 15	Superstitions re: the Newborn	114
Chapter 16	Advice for the New Parents	123
Chapter 17	Dangers to Mum & Baby	133
Chapter 18	Charms of Protection	140
Chapter 19	Religious Protection	158

PART V	BABYCARE	
Chapter 20	Naming Baby	166
Chapter 21	Babycare Superstitions	170
Chapter 22	Grooming Baby	184
Chapter 23	Remedies & Charms re: Baby's Ailments	192

PART I
CONCEPTION

Conception

CHAPTER 1
GENERAL SUPERSTITIONS

WEDDING RELATED BELIEFS

~ Coins were put in the Bride's shoe to placate Diana, the Goddess of Chastity, so the Bride could lose her virginity and conceive. *Ancient Greece*
~ Rain on your wedding day means you will have many children. *Italy*
~ Snow on your wedding day is likewise associated with fertility.
~ A baby boy, placed in the lap of a Bride, blesses her with future sons. *Turkey*
~ The Bride should kiss a baby's head at her wedding to bring her swift conception.
~ If Baby's first trip out-of-doors is to visit newlyweds, the newlyweds will soon have a baby of their own. *German Pennsylvania USA*
~ Two bottles of champagne are tied together and kept, so the couple will celebrate their first anniversary with the birth of their first child. *Russia*
~ A bottle of champagne from the reception is saved to 'wet the baby's head' at the christening. *Ireland*
~ Untie all knots before the wedding to encourage conception. *Scotland*
~ A barren woman should not be invited to the wedding, as her bad luck may rub off on the Bride. *India*
~ A red string is tied around the Bride's body; and when the wedding is over, she must breathe out so as to break the string. This procedure is sure to prevent difficult births in the future for her. *Estonia*[1]
~ If a Groom smiles a lot at his wedding, his first child will be a daughter. *Korea*
~ White storks, pomegranates, fish, fowl, wheat and midwives were all popular illustrations on wedding stationary, pastries and bridal veils, expressing the couple's wish for children. *Jewish* [2]
~ The Groom threw a fish at his Bride's feet in a fertility rite. *Libyan Jews* [2]
~ A bride jumps over a platter with a large fish on it, to shouts of blessing such as, 'may you multiply like fish'. *Jewish custom from the Balkans*[2]
~ Meeting a nun or a monk on your Wedding Day foretells barrenness.
~ The Bride 'walks with the sun' to her wedding (east to west on the south side of the church) to ensure her fertility, since the sun and fertility are associated. She then circles the Church three times 'sunwise' for luck. *Scotland*
~ During the marriage fertility rite known as 'pouring water on the hands,' the Bride and Groom's little fingers of their right hands are tied together with a white thread. The father of the bride then ritualistically pours water, a symbol of fertility, from a golden pitcher onto the thread. *Sri Lanka*

Conception

~ The word 'Bride' is derived from the name 'St. Bridget', who was the Christian version of the Irish Goddess of Fertility, Brid. ***Ireland***
~ As the Bride exits the church, onlookers break an egg to grant her many children with easy labours each time. ***Russia***
~ The moon is particularly associated with fertility. Bridal ornaments for the head and neck often represent the moon's phase in its first quarter; and it's customary to call out after newlyweds, 'Increase, O Moon.' ***Sweden***[3]
~ If a cat sneezes near the bride on her wedding day, it will bring her good luck and fertility.
~ Having the family cat or dog at a wedding grants fertility to the newlyweds.
~ The Bride's father, on the eve before his daughter leaves him, takes sugarcane from the marsh, chews it, and spits its juice onto his daughter's stomach. The sugarcane symbolises children, and is placed under the marital bed as a fertility charm. ***The Dem. Rep. of Congo***[4]
~ The Bride should pray under her wedding canopy for an infertile woman's fertility. ***Jewish***
~ As the Bride arrives home for the first time after the wedding, the fence on both sides of the entrance are pulled down, so she may drive in swiftly without obstruction. This is so her confinement (labour and the post-partum period) will come off quickly and easily. ***Estonia***[1]
~ The virgin bride should first be deflowered by a stone phallus symbolising the god Shiva. Then a fertile marriage will result. ***India***
~ Before the wedding, locks of hair were given to the goddess, Artemis, who was associated with menstruation and childbirth. ***Ancient Greece***
~ A broom used at the wedding ceremony brings fertility. ***Pagan***
~ When the Bride is fetched in, she must wear no chains or bells, but be led in in solemn silence; else she'll have restless, noisy children. ***Estonia***[1]
~ Cowrie shells are traditionally worn in a bride's necklace, and used to trim her wedding dress and headpiece to encourage her fertility. ***Africa***
~ It's usual to fast while marrying. Those who fail to fast without mighty motives will only get mute children. ***France***[1]
~ The Groom runs off with his bride. If the Bride is pregnant by the time her family catches up with them, the couple is considered married. If she isn't, her family drags her back home. The couple will run off repeatedly until the Bride conceives, or the Bride's mother decides the couple can remain together. ***Aborigine Australia***
~ The 'Best Man' cuts a small piece off a whole loaf, butters it, and puts it in the Bride's mouth so her children will have small, smooth mouths. ***Estonia***[1]
~ If the Groom ties the Bride's garters for her on her wedding day, she'll have easy labours. ***Germany*** [1]
~ The Bride's father, just before she leaves to live with her husband, takes

some white kaolin symbolising fertility passed on from his ancestors, and rubs it onto his daughter's stomach to bless her fertility. ***The Dem. Rep. of Congo***[4]
~ Breaking a coconut, pottery or an egg against a wall while facing Mecca are all considered symbolic of the hymen breaking leading to conception. The noise also confuses evil spirits, stopping them from harming the Bride's fertility. ***India, Russia & Iraq***
~ The common greeting to a new bride among some tribes is, 'May thou bear twelve children with him.' ***Africa***
~ In the wedding ride, the driver may not turn the horses, nor rein them in; or the marriage will be childless. ***Germany***[1]
~ When they see a suitor arrive on horseback, they hasten to undo his saddle-girth to ease childbirth in his possible future wife. ***Estonia***[1]
~ The word 'Honeymoon' originates from the times when the man captured his bride and hid her from her parents for one 'moon' cycle (month). During that time the couple drank a mixture of honey and wine, to increase their fertility.
~ Honey wine called 'Bunratty Meade' is traditionally drunk at weddings to promote virility. Couples also drank it from special goblets for a month following the wedding. ***Ireland***
~ Young girls carried wheat before the bride in the marriage procession, symbolising the wish the marriage would be fruitful. ***UK***
~ The Bride-to-be is given a pre-wedding dish of wheat representing fertility. ***Czech Republic***
~ Nuts were offered to the Bride and Groom as they left the church as fertility blessings. ***Ancient Rome & UK***
~ The Bride and Groom dance around Poitou's large walnut tree so the Bride will produce an abundance of future milk for her baby. ***France***
~ A husked coconut is split as the newlyweds descend from the pedestal. The manner in which the coconut halves fall apart predicts the couple's total number of children, and what their sexes will be. ***Sri Lanka***
~ If a wedding pair coming out of the Church meet a girl first, their first child will be a daughter; if a boy, a son; if a boy and girl together, they shall have twins. ***Germany***[1]
~ January is Hera's month, who was the Protectress of Wives and Fertility. January was thus a popular time for weddings. ***Ancient Greece***
~ May marriages were unlucky. Women marrying in May would be childless; or, if they had children, their firstborn would be an idiot, or have some other physical deformity.[5]
~ June's namesake is Juno, the goddess of woman, who resided over childbirth. She blessed all marriages taking place in her month. ***Ancient Rome***
~ It's unlucky to marry during the waning of the moon because the marriage

will be childless. Ideally, marry during the waxing of the moon, that is when 'the moon grows and the tide flows'. ***Orkney Islands*** [6]
~ According to fishermen, it brings bad luck and infertility to get married when the fish aren't biting. ***Scotland & Cornwall UK***

WEDDING FLOWERS

~ Two little flower girls scattered flowers before the bride, symbolising the marriage would be fruitful. ***UK***
~ Rose petals are thrown before the bride as she walks down the aisle to ward-off evil spirits below the ground and to grant fertility.
~ Yellow rose petals are thrown before the bride to grant fertility.
~ Bridal bouquets were a mixture of flowers and herbs. The flowers were symbolic amongst other things of fertility, and the strong smelling herbs repelled all evil. ***Medieval Europe***
~ The newlyweds wore floral garlands signifying a wish for fertility. Brides also carried bunches of herbs under their wedding veils as fertility symbols. ***Ancient Rome***
~ Brides wore mistletoe in their garlands to promote fertility. ***Switzerland***
~ Orange Blossoms represent fertility and were often used at weddings for this reason. Juno, Goddess of maternity and childbirth, was said to have given them to Jupiter on her wedding day. ***Ancient Rome***
~ If it rains on the bridal wreath, the couple will be rich and fertile. ***Germany*** [1]

WEDDING CAKE

~ The wedding cake is actually a fertility cake, as large, sweet cakes have long been associated with fertility in Christian tradition. ***Roman Catholic***
~ The wedding cake was originally made from many small wheat cakes (in Scotland, oat cakes) that were thrown over the Bride's head like confetti to bless her fertility. This evolved to crumbling or even breaking the cake over the Bride's head.
~ A plate of cake was flung over the Bride's head as she returned from the church, and fertility omens were read from the manner is which the plate broke. The number of broken bits of plate indicated the number of children she would have. ***England***
~ Early wedding cakes were flat and round, containing fruit and nuts symbolising fertility. ***UK***
~ Traditionally, the bottom layer of a wedding cake represents the couple as a family, and the top layer represents them as a couple. Each layer in between represents a child they will have.
~ The top tier should be an Irish whiskey cake, to be saved for the christening of the couple's first baby. ***Ireland***
~ The Bride must cut the first piece of cake or she'll have a childless marriage.

CONFETTI

~ Throwing confetti originates from the custom of showering a couple with grain and nuts (life-giving seeds) to transfer the seeds' fertility onto the couple. *Pagan*

~ The walnut was associated with Juno, the goddess of women and marriage. Walnuts were therefore thrown at the Bride and Groom for fertility. *Ancient Rome*

~ Nuts were offered to the Bride and Groom as they left the church as fertility blessings. *Ancient Rome & UK*

~ While the couple are still kneeling at the foot of the altar, a rain of nuts is poured over their heads and down their backs. *Gaillac: France*

~ As a Bride leaves Church, an elderly woman presents her with a little bag containing hazel nuts to enhance her fertility. *Devon*

~ As grains and nuts representing new life and plenty were thrown at the Newlyweds, onlookers shouted, 'Be fertile and increase!' *Jewish Custom in Europe & Asia* [2]

~ The Groom's parents throw nuts and plums to a bride after her wedding. If the Bride picks up some nuts, she'll have many sons. *Korea*

~ As the Bride and Groom walk down the street, onlookers throw not only rice, but larger items as well, such as pots and pans. *Ireland*

~ Rice was thrown as confetti in the UK, India & USA; Wheat in France, Germany & Holland; Bread, wheat or salt in Italy; fruit and nuts in Ancient Greece; Nuts in France, Sugared almonds in Italy, Eggs is some parts of Europe, red dates in Korea, and figs, dates and raisins in Morocco.

~ The shoe is a symbol of life, especially as shown in productivity and fertility. Hence old shoes are thrown after a bride, the Jewish crying, 'Increase and multiply'. The following nursery rhyme can be traced back to this early mythology:

'There was an old woman who lived in a shoe,
Who had so many children she didn't know what to do.' [7]

~ A handful of sand was scattered before the Bride & Groom to echo the promise given to Abraham, the Father of the Jews, 'I will make your descendants as numerous as the grains of sand on the seashore.' *Jewish*

WEDDING PRESENTS

~ Rose quartz is traditionally given to brides to promote pregnancies and discourage miscarriages.

~ Mango leaves are presented at weddings to bless the couple with sons. *India*

~ Wedding guests are given beautifully decorated hardboiled eggs, symbolic of the Newlyweds' wish for children. *Malaysia*

~ The gift of five almonds represents health, wealth, happiness, long life, and fertility. *Europe*

Conception

~ The person who gives the third gift to be opened at wedding will soon have a baby.
~ The Newlyweds are wrapped in a gift of a batik cloth called a 'selendang'. This symbolises the hope for the couple to have children, as the selendang is traditionally used to carry babies. *Malaysia*
~ Traditional wedding steins had acorn-shaped thumb-lifts, the acorn being symbolic of fertility. *Germany*
~ In Holland & Switzerland, a pine tree, symbolic of luck and fertility, is planted outside the couple's home as a wedding present. In Norway, two small pine trees are placed on either side of the Newlywed's front door until they have a baby.
~ Terracotta elephants are traditional wedding gifts, as elephants are associated with rain, which makes the fields fertile. *India*

THE BRIDAL BED

~ In Cyprus, a chubby baby boy is rolled up and down the marital bed before the wedding night so the couple will be blessed with boys. In the Czech Republic, a baby is similarly laid on the bed to bless the marriage with children.
~ A woman still producing breast milk should prepare the marital bed to encourage the newlyweds' fertility. *Scotland*
~ A hen that was a prolific layer was tied to the bed on the first night in the hope its fertility would be passed onto the couple. *Ireland*
~ A honeymoon bed sheet should be blue to ensure the husband's virility and the granting of future sons. *Mexico*
~ The marital bed is traditionally arranged by an elderly couple who leave symbols of fertility such as rice and sesame seeds between its sheets. *Thailand*

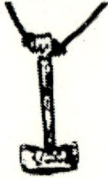

The Hammer of Thor (Mjölner) is the symbol for Thor, the god of thunder and lightning, who was the friend and protector of all humans. According to legend, the hammer was forged by dwarves knowledgeable in magic and brought to Asgård, the home of the gods, as a gift to Thor. The hammer symbol stands for protection against evil forces and is a fertility symbol. Hammer symbols were put in the bed of newlyweds to protect their fertility. *Sweden* [8]
~ The couple's parents often tucked a fish between the newlyweds' sheets to ensure fertility. *Oriental Jewish*

~ The Scottish place a willow branch beneath the newlyweds' bed to promote pregnancy. Pagans place a broom.
~ As the blood of the hymen was greatly feared, the Best Man was sometimes expected to consummate the marriage on behalf of the groom, to ensure no bad luck or evil spirits could destroy the couple's fertility!
~ Friends of the Newlyweds' burst into the bridal chamber and offered the couple soup from the chamber pot to give them strength and fertility. **Languedoc France**

OTHER CONCEPTION & FERTILITY BELIEFS

~ If someone with a baby leaves an article of baby clothing at your home, or throws away a used nappy the next time she visits, this will bless you with the patter of tiny feet. *USA*
~ The childless should adopt, and then the woman will fall pregnant with one of her own. *UK*
~ If a woman puts two spoons into her saucer, she'll have ginger twins. *UK*
~ A man's brothers have conjugal rights to the bride as she is viewed as being married to the family. If she becomes pregnant a 'Pursutpimi Ceremony' is performed to determine paternity. After a discussion amongst the brothers, the chosen man is presented with a bow and arrow under a Kiaz tree. All further children borne by the woman are then considered that man's, even if he dies, unless another ceremony is performed. *Todras Tribe India*
~ What a woman sees just before and during conception greatly affects her baby. Looking at certain things can mould Baby's looks or character. Mum should look only at pleasant things; if she sees something unpleasant, she must ritually cleanse herself right away. *Jewish*[2]
~ Anything other than the 'Missionary' sexual position produces savage babies. *Victorian UK*
~ Throw a tablecloth from a christening dinner over a barren wife to make her pregnant. *Germany* [1]
~ Mingling with pregnant women or even pregnant animals, makes their fertility rub off on you. Steer clear of all barren animals and women though, as it works both ways. *India & Jewish*
~ Accidentally stepping in a child's shadow will result in a woman becoming pregnant.
~ According to Irish legend, if a woman dreams that a spark falls into her mouth or lap, it's the soul coming to her child. In Yorkshire, a falling star is a child's soul coming into the world.[9]
~ The Americans believe rocking an empty cradle will soon fill it with child. In Caithness (Scotland) they say, 'If you rock the cradle empty, you shall have babies plenty.'
~ Ritually whipping young girls encourages fertility in the whole tribe.

Ancient Romans, Ancient Greeks & Druids
~ Use the principal of finding a 'scapegoat': that is, find a fertile animal, place your hand on it, and ritually transfer your infertility onto it. ***Jewish & Pagan***
~ A holy well on May Island was a popular destination for infertile women to make pilgrimages to in the Middle Ages to pray for a cure. ***Scotland***
~ In the Philippines, knitting baby things before you're pregnant is bad luck; it may prevent you from getting pregnant, or make a sickly future baby. Likewise, the Jewish believe it's very unlucky to give names to a yet-to-be conceived child.
~ Hugging certain trees grants fertility. According to whether the woman hugs the east or west side, affects the sex of the baby. ***Maori***
~ Place your nightgown on a fruitful tree on St George's Eve in order to conceive. ***South Slavonia***
~ Sitting on cold surfaces causes infertility. ***Russia***
~ Telling others of your plans to have a child risks 'The Evil Eye' (see evil 139). This can scupper your plans entirely.
~ A barren woman is suspected of having had sex with a vampire or spirit before marriage. ***Eastern European Romany Gypsy*** [7]
~ A 'Baloma' (spirit of a dead woman) sees an embryo; picks it up, and places it in another woman's womb while she is bathing. Mum-to-be will feel as if a fish has bitten her, when in fact, it's the Baloma placing an embryo into her. Unmarried girls deem it much better precaution to avoid bathing at high tide, than to be chaste. ***Trobriand Islanders Melanesia*** [10]
~ The being, Anjea, causes conception by putting mud babies into women's wombs. ***Australia***
~ The 'mother-sheaf' of corn is made into the likeness of a pregnant woman and given to the farmer's wife, in the belief that she who binds the last sheaf will have a child within one year. ***Breton***
~ To find out how many children you'll have, cut an apple in half and count how many seeds are inside, or count the number of Xs in the palm of your right hand, or pick a dandelion that has gone to seed and blow the seeds into the wind. The number of seeds left on the stem represents the number of your children.
~ Hang your wedding ring from a strand of your hair. Rub the ring up and down your index finger a couple of times and then hold it above the top of your outstretched right hand. The number of times the ring swings around in a circle before stopping will predict how many children you'll have.
~ On Halloween, blindfolded girls plucked heads of oats and counted the number of grains to find out how many children they would have. Alternately, they dropped egg-white into a glass of water and counted the number of times it divided. ***Scotland*** [11]

TIME OF CONCEPTION

~ Conceiving at midday or midnight produces a bad-tempered foetus.
~ Don't begin anything on a Monday, for the project will not live to be a week old. **France**
~ Never conceive on a Friday as it's a terrible day to start anything. **UK**
~ In the Celtic calendar, the first twenty days of January are in the month of 'Beth', the birch tree, which represents beginnings, creation and fertility. This month is dedicated to the Mother Goddess, and is said to be a particularly potent time to conceive. **Celtic**
~ May Day (the festival of 'Beltane') is a very fertile time and is an excellent time to conceive. Huge bonfires were lit in honour of the fertile Sun God, and homes were adorned with flowers to bring in the fertilising powers of nature. The crowning of the May Queen, Morris Dancing, and dancing around a garlanded Maypole are all ancient fertility rites. **Celtic**
~ The dew of May morning was renowned for healing all varieties of illnesses, including infertility. Other May morning healing rituals involve bathing in the waters from the various Holy Wells. **Cornwall** [12]
~ Make love when the tide is coming in, not going out, so the tide does not wash away the man's seed with it.
~ Imbolc (a.k.a. Oimelc, St. Brigid's Day or Candlemas) celebrated on or around the first day of February, symbolises the first stirring of life after winter, and the creative powers of nature and the fertility God, Cernunnos. **Celtic**

SIGNS A BABY IS COMING

~ If a child bends over forward and looks between his legs, he is 'looking fi deh bredda' (looking for his brother or sister). This means his mother is going to have another baby soon. **Belize**
~ A whistling girl will surely have a bastard child. Therefore, mothers of fine breeding forbid their daughters the 'pleasure' of whistling. **German Pennsylvania USA**
~ If a woman bakes a cake and the middle of the cake sinks, then she's pregnant. **Belize**
~ If your nose itches, someone you know will have a baby. **Japan**
~ If your right eye twitches, there will soon be a birth in the family.
~ When family members have cravings for food they normally don't eat, the cravings are taken to be signs that someone else in the family is pregnant. **Pacific Islands**
~ If an apron falls off, a baby is due. Likewise, 'Spoon falls, baby calls'. **UK**
~ To dream about pomegranates, represents fertility. Dreaming of a black and white cat means luck with children; possibly the birth of a child. If you dream of a death or wedding, it's said to be a sign of a birth. If you dream about

rabbits you'll soon breed yourself. If you dream of fish, it's a sign someone is pregnant.
~ If a man pours tea for a woman, she'll have a baby.
~ If a gypsy woman in Transylvania wishes to know whether she is pregnant, she must stand for nine evenings at a crossroads with an axe or hammer, which she must urinate on and bury there. If the axe is found rusty after being dug up nine mornings later, it's a sign that she's pregnant. ***Gypsy*** [7]

Chapter 2
Charms & Amulets

~ An amber stone found on the seashore brings Mother Earth's powers to whoever finds it.
~ On Midsummer's Eve, pick St John's Wort while naked to get pregnant. ***Pagan***
~ If you want to conceive, try on the shoes of a woman who has just given birth. ***UK***
~ Barren women eat grass from the grave in which a pregnant woman has been buried and then chant to receive the dead woman's fertility. ***Hungarian Gypsy*** [7]
~ A charm in the shape of baby feet or baby shoes encourages conception. ***USA***
~ A 'yad' necklace portraying an open hand has Kabbalistic (mystical) powers to ward off evil and encourage conception. ***Jewish***
~ The 'Figa' symbol (a hand with the thumb between the first two fingers) was originally a fertility symbol. ***Brazil***
~ When rug making, weaving with the colour brown enhances fertility. ***Asia***
~ The mother stands upstream, and her youngest daughter stands naked downstream. As the mother dips herself in the steam, her daughter washes herself in the water flowing down from her mother, and drinks some of it to internalise her mother's fertility. The mother cuts a fertility string from her waist and allows it to float downstream, telling her daughter to tie it around her waist, thereby passing on her fertility. The mother then floats leaves from the Mushie tree downstream to her daughter saying, 'These Mushie leaves will enable you to be flexible during childbirth and to give birth without difficulty. Wear them around your waist.' ***Congo*** [4]
~ Standing angel statues by the bed brings fertility. ***USA***
~ A grouping of three statues in the bedroom 'home corner' symbolises the wish for two to become three, as a type of Feng-Shui. ***UK & USA***
~ The woman drinks water in which her husband has cast hot coals, or better still has spit, saying, 'Where I am flame, be thou the coals, Where I am rain, be thou the water!' ***Romany Gypsy*** [7]
~ Burning green candles enhances a link with the Mother Goddess, inducing fertility. Key words such as 'pregnancy' and 'baby' can be carved into the candles. Lighting the candle and then chanting the words, draws powers into the words. After the power has been raised, it's released into the Universe, where the words start taking effect. ***Wiccan Magic***
~ Every May, scores of childless couples dance an ancient fertility dance,

while pushing wooden carts filled with images of the Virgin of the Fishing Raft to whom they are appealing for children. ***Obando: Philippines***
~ In ancient times, Belly Dancing was performed by priestesses and was considered an important part of fertility rituals performed to placate gods. Its movements were associated with the movements of labour. In the 19th Century, belly dancing was performed among women only. ***Iraq***
~ A birth altar with candles, eggs, seeds, herbs, charms, statues, baby clothes etc. acts as a focus to draw in fertile creative energy from the Universe. ***Pagan***
~ When a mother looses her first child when he is still very young, he is buried under her bed to keep him safe so he will return to her. If the woman does not conceive again for a long time, the parents exhume the child's body and the mother takes one of the bones from the baby's skeleton and wears it around her waist to restore her fertility. She then prays, asking her dead child to return to her womb. ***Congo*** [4]

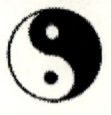   Yin/Yang Symbol: Helps to balance and harmonise sexual energies. ***China***
~ Certain churches are adorned with wax figures of babies, put there by mothers to pray for a successful pregnancy. ***Eastern Europe***
~ Because it's a product of the sea, or the 'all generating moisture,' and because of its shape, the seashell is an emblem of women. The shell also represents the Moon and fertility. The shell is historically the world's most popular amulet, opposed to barrenness and all evil.
~ A whalebone 'Tiki' amulet represents the fertility of the first man on Earth. A charm for male virility, it's worn on a chain around the neck. ***Polynesia***
~ An amulet with the scripture from Exodus 23:26: 'No woman in your land shall miscarry or be barren' acts as a fertility blessing. ***Jewish***
~ Fatima, the Creatoress and source of fate, was the Moon Goddess in pre-Islamic Arabia. Her hand symbol is a protective amulet, and also a fertility charm.
~ Mermaids are symbols of fertility found in many culture's creation myths.
~ The Rod of the Greek God, Asclepius, is a symbol of healing and fertility. Asclepius's Rod consists of a serpent entwined around a staff, shedding its skin in a symbol of rebirth and fertility. ***Ancient Greece***
~ The pregnancy and childbirth goddess, Hathor, known as the 'Great Menat', used the Menat, a heavy beaded necklace with a crescent shaped front to channel her powers over life, fertility, birth, and rebirth. For this reason, the image of the Menat was a fertility symbol. Hathor's attention was attracted by using a Sistrum, a sacred rattle that brought fertility and banished evil spirits. The sistrum consisted of a wooden or metal frame fitted with loose strips of

metal and disks which jingled when moved. *Ancient Egypt*
~ The Ankh was the Egyptian cross of life and symbolised life power. When worn or carried, the ankh promoted fertility. The gods are often seen offering the 'The Breath of Life' by holding an ankh to someone's lips. Some people now believe the ankh represents the union of male and female sexual symbols: the circle at the top representing the female sexual organ, the stump at the bottom, the male organ, and the crossed line, the children of their union.
Ancient Egypt

BROOMS
~ The broom is an ancient fertility symbol. Some brooms were made of Ash or Birch, a sacred wood renowned for its powers of fertility. Jumping over a broom on Beltane (May Day) brought fertility. *Celtic*
~ The broom sweeps away bad luck and evil spells causing infertility. *Voodoo*
~ A charm in the shape of a broom enhances fertility. *Pagan*
~ A man hit with a broom becomes impotent unless he retaliates seven times with the same broom. *Nigeria*

CORDS OR RIBBONS
~ A red cord worn around the wrist has kabbalistic (mystical) powers to ward off evil and encourage fertility. *Jewish*
~ Each partner should wear a cord for a month, beginning at the woman's most fertile time. At the end of the month, the two cords should be tied together, symbolising two beings creating a third, and this should be placed beneath the marital bed. *Pagan*
~ A woman wears a red cord, a symbol bringing together both a good life and fertility, around the wrist of her right hand. *Congo*[4]
~ Put a red cord through your diary at your fertile time. *Pagan*
~ A pink cord should be worn if a girl is desired, and a blue cord should be worn for a boy.

FERTILITY DOLLS & STATUES
~ The Corn Dolly is a fertility symbol, and hung over the marital bed, or placed within an empty crib, blesses the house with children. *Celtic*
~ The statues of men with extremely large phallus are widely sold in Middle Eastern lands. For many, these are not just fun souvenirs but potent male virility symbols.
~ An infertile woman takes a wooden Akua'ba doll, blessed by a priest, and treats it like a real baby, carrying it with her constantly. She tends the doll until she has a baby of her own. After the child is born, the doll is placed in a household shrine. The Akua'ba doll is named in honour of a barren woman named Akua who did this and eventually conceived and gave birth to a child. *Ashanti Tribe Ghana*
~ 'Gosho dolls', clay dolls of white-skinned, large-headed chubby little boys,

were widely used as fertility charms. A gift of a Gosho doll was considered a wish for the recipient to have strong, healthy sons. ***Japan***
~ Red ochre was smeared on fertility statues symbolising blood, a life-force. Other charms were smeared with actual menstrual blood. ***Ancient Mesopotamia***
~ From childhood, girls wear fertility dolls around their necks or on their hips as a plea to the gods for many children. ***Turkana People: Kenya***

GEMS AND STONES
~ Reuben, the High Priest, was said to have helped the Matriarch, Rachel, conceive, and his stone in the High Priest's breastplate was red. Therefore, the belief evolved that red stones could cure infertility. Amulet rings were set with ruby with various inscriptions such as 'Joseph is a fruitful vine', ruby was crushed into a powder and mixed with wine for the infertile woman to drink, and even today, infertile women will borrow red stones from the Rabbi's wife to help them conceive. ***Jewish*** [2]
~ Pink Jasper and Rose Quartz are fertility stones.
~ Turquoise, Lapis Lazuli and Feldspar's blue colour symbolises fertility, luck and protection against the 'Evil Eye'. ***Ancient Egypt***

HORNS
~ Horns and antlers are symbols of virility. ***Celtic***
~ The golden horn is an amulet against evil and promotes male virility and sex appeal. ***Italy***
~ The 'Horn of Plenty' charm gives abundance in all areas of life, including fertility.
~ A deer horn placed under the bed brings fertility.

RUNES
~ Runes are an ancient form of European writing. They are also potent magical symbols, invoking spiritual powers. Traditionally, runes are hand-carved on wood, (the wood, a living soul, becoming part of the magic) and fertility runes were stained with menstrual blood. Nowadays, runic symbols are also engraved on stone and metal and placed or painted on all manner of objects.
~ Carve a fertility rune onto some cheese and then eat the cheese to internalise the magic.
~ Wear a rune as a fertility charm around the neck.

Berkano Rune: associated with the Nordic fertility Goddess, Freya, this rune is said to increase female sexual energies and fertility.

Jera Rune (a.k.a. Jara): A fertility rune connected to Frey and Freya symbolising the cycle of sowing and harvesting: so what is 'sowed' by the man will be 'harvested' in the woman.

or **Ingwaz Rune** (a.k.a. Ng and Ing): associated with the Nordic fertility god, Ing, this rune can be used to increase fertility in both sexes but is particularly good for men.

~ A fertility symbol tattoo can be applied to the man or woman with henna or permanent dye. The fertility charm can also be drawn on the body with saliva, blood, vaginal fluid or semen.

~ Lay fertility runes under the marital bed. (It's important the runes are the correct way up at all times, otherwise the opposite energy could be invoked to that desired.)

STANDING STONES

~ Contact with Standing Stones causes barren women to have children. The Celts left a small offering on the stone. Similar rites were practised at megalithic monuments. The spirits of the dead were expected to assist these rites, or even to incarnate themselves in the children born as a result of resorting to these stones. [13]

~ In Brittany and Cornwall, the woman passes through the hole of a dolmen (a naturally pierced stone) to cure her infertility. In Ireland, many dolmens are known as 'Diarmaid and Grainne's beds', places where these legendary eloping lovers slept. Therefore, these stones have fertility powers and are visited by barren women. [13]

~ Women dance naked around the stones and rub against them in the hope of becoming mothers. ***Brittany France*** [9]

~ Girls slide down the stone of St Samson, and if they can reach the bottom without a hitch, they will be happy mothers when married. ***Dinan: France*** [9]

~ The Standing Stone is a symbol of male fertility and power, used as a phallic symbol, marking a centre of energy. The man should place his hands upon the stone to ask for virility. ***Ireland***

CHAPTER 3
RELIGIOUS BELIEFS

~ Attempt to earn God's favour by undertaking charity work to mark the occasion of trying to conceive. *Jewish*
~ One of the most popular gravesites in Israel for infertile women to pray for conception at, is the grave of the Matriarch Rachel (who also struggled with conception). *Jewish*
~ Before sex, prayer is recited to protect any fertilised egg from the devil. The Qarina come into the world from the time the child is conceived. Therefore, during sex, 'bismillah' is said to prevent any child that might be conceived from being overcome by their devilish qarina (see page 134). *Moslem*
~ The couple should pray for protection from Lilith, the fabled first wife of Adam, and now a female demon that lurks in the marriage bed to conceive demons from sperm. The couple should pull the sheets over their heads for one hour after sex to keep Lilith away from any spilt semen. *Jewish* [2]
~ When a woman is childless, a 'making the curse fly away' ceremony is performed. A sacrifice of three grasshoppers is offered up to the gods. Then a swallow is set free, with a prayer that the curse of infertility may fly away with the bird. *The Bataks Sumatra* [14]
~ Seven spirits cause infertility. According to a magical book given to King Solomon, using potions such as wolf's womb and bear spleen can protect against these spirits. *Jewish*
~ Some Roman Catholic women use Baby Jesus statues to specifically pray to for a child. Others prefer to pray to statues of the Virgin Mary. *Slavic*

THE FERTILITY GODS & GODDESSES

~ I have included many of the ancient deities, as recently there has been renewed interest and worship of them amongst 'New Age' groups, Pagans and Wiccans. The deities may have other roles not related to fertility which for simplicity's sake I have not included here.

Ai Apaec: The fertility god who could assume the form of a tomcat. *Peru*
Ala: *Nigeria*
Ama no Uzume: goddess whose dance became a fertility rite. *Japan*
Anat: *Canaan*
Anu: Mother Earth Goddess *Ireland*
Aphrodite: Goddess of sexual passion, representing fertility through the act of sexual intercourse. *Ancient Greece*
Arianrhod: (a.k.a. 'Silver Wheel' and the 'High Fruitful Mother') One face of the Mother Goddess associated with fertility and reincarnation. *Wales*
Aritimi: *Ancient Rome*

Baby Lore

Ashur: *Assyria*
Astarte: *Ancient Egypt*
Althaea: birth goddess *Ancient Greece*
Baal: *Canaan*
Backlum Chaam: God of male sexuality. *Mayan*
Bat: *Ancient Egypt*
Bel: fertility and healing god *Ireland and Wales*
Bendis: female fertility goddess. *Ancient Greece*
Bona Dea: *Ancient Rome*
Bright Mother: the ovulating goddess.
Brigit: the goddess of women, healing, and fertility. The Roman Catholic St Brigid seems to have taken on most of Brigit's characteristics. *Ireland*
Cernunnos: (a.k.a. 'The Horned One' or 'Lord of the Forest') Fertility god usually shown in the company of fertile stags and ram-horned snakes in a forest setting. Cernunnos goes through a yearly cycle of birth, death and rebirth. The first sign of his rebirth is the lambs born at Imbolc (1st February). He marries the Mother Goddess at Beltaine (1st May) when the powers of nature are at their peak, and then dies at the time of the first harvest at Lughnasadh (1st August), as the barley and wheat are cut down. *Celtic*
Chauturopayini: fertility goddess *Hindi*
Chalchihuitlicue: creative goddess *Aztec*
Chicomecoatl: fertility goddess *Mayan*
Cybele: *Ancient Rome*
Danu (Dana); The Celtic mother goddess who was often depicted in triple form, because three was a sacred number, and multiplication of an image by three increased its power. *Ireland*
Dionysus: fertility God *Ancient Greece*
Earth Mother: always depicted as being pregnant
Erce: Mother Earth and 'Fruitful Womb' in Old English
Fauna: *Ancient Rome*
Fecunditas: *Ancient Rome*
Frigg: the wife of Odin (the king of the gods). Frigg made men fertile and invoking her name brought babies. *Scandinavia*
Freya: goddess of sexual activity. *Scandinavia*
Gefjon: one of Frigg's handmaidens who was associated with fertility in both men and nature. To ensure crop fertility, a strip of ground was ploughed in her name before the entire field each year. *Scandinavia*
Ghede: *Voudoun*
Hera: The Queen of the gods who ruled over maternity. *Ancient Greece*
Hun Hunahpu: A fertility god, so fertile that when his severed head was placed on a barren gourd it immediately began to bear fruit. *Mayan*

Conception

Isis: The Great Mother *Ancient Egypt*

Ixchel: (meaning 'rainbow') The Weaver or Creatrix goddess who ruled childbirth, lunar cycles, and pregnancy. She was normally represented as a gnarled old woman, with a snake headband and skirt embroidered with crossbones. The rite of passage into womanhood required making a clay image of Ixchel, travelling to her temple on the sacred Isla Mujeres (Isle of Women) and performing a ritualistic breaking of her image. *Mayan*

Juno Sospita: One of the many faces of Juno (queen of the gods) who was often called upon by infertile women. *Ancient Rome*

Ilamatecuhtli: fertility goddess *Aztec*

Kahmden: mother goddess *Hindu*

Khnum: called the 'Father of Fathers and the Mother of Mothers', his name means 'to create'. Khnum fashioned the bodies and spirits of every child born on his potter's wheel. He also gave health to the newborn. *Ancient Egypt*

Kokopelli: 'the seed bringer' - childless women begged him to stay and play his flute to bless them with children. *Native American*

Maia: *Anatolian*

Oestre: fertility goddess *Anglo-Saxon*

Tellus Mater: *Celtic*

Pukkeenegak: *Eskimo*

Hutu (Hou-T'u): *China*

Lono: *Polynesian*

Macha: Fertility goddess mainly connected with male virility. *Ireland*

Mahueret: Egyptian goddess of beginnings *Ancient Egypt*

Min: god of male virility, depicted with an erect penis, married to Quetesh, the fertility goddess. Min was honoured in the Pharaoh's coronation rites to ensure the production of a male heir. *Ancient Egypt*

Mnewer: *Ancient Egypt*

Mutinus: *Ancient Rome*

Narayana: God born from the primordial egg whose name is sometimes associated with the egg itself. *Hindu*

Osiris: *Ancient Egypt*

Pan: represented male virility. *Ancient Greece*

Quetesh: fertility goddess. *Ancient Egypt*

Rhea: *Ancient Greece*

Sahur: *Phoenician*

Shakti: Goddess of creative power *Hindu*

Shiva: God of fertility, medicine, and sexual love *Hindu*

Sri-Laksmi: the Lotus Goddess. Her power over fertility and abundance is even older than Uma's. *Hindu*

Tlaloc: the great rain and fertility god. *Mayan*

Turan: *Ancient Rome*
Uma: Goddess of womanhood, particularly childbirth. *Hindu*
Venus: fertility goddess *Ancient Rome*
Vitumnus: God who gave life to the foetus *Ancient Rome*
Xipe Tot^c: 'Our Lord of the Flayed One' - A phallic fertility god *Aztec*

ROMAN CATHOLIC SAINTS

Patron Saint to Conceive, against Sterility, Barrenness, Conception Difficulties;
Agatha, Anne, Anthony of Padua, Casilda of Toledo, Felicity, Fiacre, Francis of Paola, Giles, Henry II, Margaret of Antioch, Medard, Philomena, Rita of Cascia, Theobald Roggeri
Patron Saint of Desperate, Impossible or Lost causes; Jude Thaddeus, Gregory Thaumaturgus, Philomena, Rita of Cascia
Patron Saint of Childless People; Anne Line, Catherine of Genoa, Gummarus, Henry II, Julian the Hospitaller
Patron Saint to have Male Children; Felicity
Patron Saint of Doctors; Cosmas, Damian, Luke the Apostle, Pantaleon, Raphael the Archangel
Patron Saints of Adopted Children; Clotilde, Thomas More, William of Rochester

Conception

CHAPTER 4
THE POWERS OF NATURE

FIRE & SUN

~ Fire keeps away evil spells or spirits that are the true cause of conception difficulties.
~ Fire is a fertility symbol. ***Sri Lanka***
~ Brigit, the mother goddess, is surrounded by fire. ***Ireland***
~ Fire is related to the fertile sun. The great fertility feast of *Bel*, the Sun, took place on May Eve. The Celts lit huge bonfires at *Beltaine*.
~ The Druids lit the *Baal-Tinne*, the holy fire of *Baal*, the Sun-god, and then drove the cattle on a path made between two fires, singing them with the flame of a lighted torch to make them fertile. In the mystic snake dance, performed at the Baal festival, the gyrations of the dancers were always westward, in the path of the sun, for the dance was part of the ancient ritual of sun worship.[15]
~ In Scandinavia, a young virgin did a fertility dance. Wearing a metal belt depicting the sun, she danced around so the rays of the sun reflected against her belt as she spun around the group throwing seed and pollen.
~ Jumping over a bonfire at the time of the summer solstice enables a woman to conceive. ***Pagan***
~ Most of the Sun Gods in every culture are strongly related to fertility, because of the obvious connection with the sun bringing life, warmth and growth to nature.
~ The sun disk symbol of Pharoah Akhenaten brings the powers of the sun, fertility and healing into one symbol. ***Ancient Egypt***

The Sun Fertility Symbol: giver of life, warmth, growth, all that is good. The rays signify the four directions. ***Native American***

The Spiral, an ancient sun symbol, can be found in many cultures; the oldest found engraved on a 24,000-year-old mammoth tooth made by Cro-Magnon hunters. This symbol was popular in Scandinavia during the

Bronze and Iron Ages, and symbolises life force, energy and the seed of life. [8]

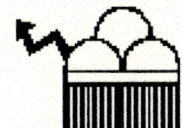 The Sun fertility symbol: the same symbol appears in many ancient cultures; e.g.: to the Native Americans it's known as the 'Whirling Logs Fertility Symbol', depicting the cyclic motion of life, seasons and the four winds. Taken from the image of a tree in a whirlwind, it's considered a powerful medicine. *Ancient Egypt*

WATER & RAIN

~ At the dawn of a New Year, a woman drops a small bundle of ritualistic items into a well before the first bucket of the year is drawn from it. The first water drawn is then kept in a small container. If, at the yearend, there's no drop in the container's water level, it's a sign that the New Year will be fertile and prosperous. *Sri Lanka*

~ In the Congo, a woman stands naked in the rain while an infertility ritualist calls on his ancestors to take away her infertility with the rainwater.[4] Pagans have a similar ritual, albeit it can only be performed on May Morning or Midsummer's night, and deities rather than ancestors are called upon.

Clouds, Rain and Lightning Fertility Symbol representing fertility. Snow is considered a greater blessing than rain. *Native American*

~ The well is a symbol of the feminine and is an entrance to the womb of the goddess. Drawing water from a well, particularly one blessed by a Saint, enhances a woman's fertility. *Ireland*

~ The river was a divinity, a source of fertility, regarded as a giver of life, health, and plenty. A fertility cult surrounded the river goddesses who were offered gifts and sacrifices. Offerings of cloth, wool, or coins were also thrown to the divinities that lived in lakes or wells (hence the tradition of throwing coins into a wishing well). If a woman is pricked with a pin, and the pin thrown into the well, her infertility will be banished into the well. *Celtic*[13]

~ The Irish crept on their hands and knees around holy wells, always westward, following the course of the sun. The ancient Persians at their sacred fountains, also always followed the sun's path.[15]

~ Certain springs at Sinuessa were believed to possess the power of preventing childlessness. *Ancient Rome* [16]

THE MOON

~ As the moon moves in twenty nine day cycles, it became strongly associated with the female menstruation cycle, fertility and childbirth.

~ The Goddesses of fertility are all strongly associated with the moon in Greek and Roman mythology. Metztli, the Aztec Goddess of the moon and childbirth, and Akna, the Aztec Goddess of motherhood, are also both associated with the moon.

~ To many ancient cultures, the crescent moon became a sacred symbol of the goddess, the feminine, and fertility.

~ The crescent moon lunar phase was said to be the best time to conceive. The horseshoe symbolises the crescent moon, which is perhaps why it came to be used in wedding ceremonies as a fertility blessing. ***Ancient Greece***

~ Wearing a piece of pink quartz shaped like a crescent moon promotes female fertility.

~ Moon-shaped amulets are particularly potent for people born under the astrological sign of Cancer, which is ruled by the moon.

~ The moon has phallic overtones. In ancient symbolism, the horns of the moon were synonymous with the horns of the ox - the ox symbolic of productiveness and fertility.

'Pray to the Moon when she is round,
Luck with you will then abound,
What you seek for shall be found,
On the sea or solid ground.' ***Romany Gypsy*** [7]

~ If a newly married woman looks at the new moon regularly, she'll deliver a son as handsome as the moon.

~ If you conceive at the full moon, you will deliver at the full moon. ***UK***

ANIMAL, BIRD & INSECT SYMBOLS & SUPERSTITIONS

- **BEARS**

~ Bears symbolise childbearing and powerful protective motherly instincts. Bear symbols are used as fertility charms. ***Pagan***

- **BEETLES**

~ The scarab beetle, Khepri, was linked to the god Khepera, a solar fertility deity. Khepera rolled the fertile ball of the sun across the heavens as the scarab beetles roll their fertile balls of dung across the ground. The scarab Beetle thus became Khepara's symbol and was depicted on all kinds of amulets and seals. ***Ancient Egypt***

~ In one version of the creation myth, a lotus flower rose out of the primeval waters of Nun, the infinite ocean of chaos. The lotus's petals parted to reveal a scarab beetle which then transformed into a boy, who wept tears that became mankind. ***Ancient Egypt***

~ Powdered scarab beetles taken in water act as modern day conception

charms. ***Egypt & Sudan***
- **BIRDS**

~ If a cockerel responds to the song of a cuckoo, a woman nearby will become pregnant. ***French***

~ When the belly-mema bird whistles, it signifies someone in the area is pregnant. ***Guyana***

~ Four magpies seen together are a sign of a forthcoming birth. ***Cornwall UK***

~ The woodpecker is a fertility symbol.

~ The peacock that dances to attract a mate when the rains come is seen as a fertility symbol, as rain makes the crops fertile. ***India***

~ As water is such a potent fertile source, all water birds become associated with fertility by default.

~ To the Native Americans, parrots carry specific prayer requests and bring blessings. Parrots are also connected with both the coming of the sun and rain, both fertility symbols, so become fertility symbols in their own right. In India, Parrots are likewise associated with fertility.

- **BULLS**

~ The Bull is an ancient fertility symbol in many cultures, particularly used to bless male virility. Some men drank powdered bull's horn to increase their virility.

~ The bull, the leader of the cattle, symbolises the herd (family or clan) and its fertility. The bull's symbol was used in a ceremony to magically join the bull's fertility with the tribe's. In Gaul, the Bull represented the Solar God who made the Earth Mother fertile. ***Celtic***

~ Bull's horns were sometimes placed around the camp to increase male virility. ***Pagan***

~ Wear a bull shaped amulet, or place one beneath the bed to increase fertility in men *and* women. The bull symbol is especially powerful for people born under the astrological sign of Taurus. ***Pagan***

- **BUTTERFLIES**

~ Butterflies are found around water and thus become associated with fertility and rebirth. ***Native American***

~ Because of its beauty and delicacy, the butterfly symbolises all that is female, including fertility.

~ If the first butterfly of the season is yellow, it's an omen of a birth. ***Brunswick Canada***

~ The dead are reborn as children who fly about as butterflies. Therefore, butterflies are signs of fertility as they bring children. ***Bavaria***

- **CATS**

~ Cats are extremely fertile, and so were adopted by various cultures as fertility symbols.

Conception

~ According to Hellenic cosmogony, the moon created the cat.[17] The cat was sacred to Diana (a.k.a. Artemis) the goddess of the moon and fertility, so therefore had some of her fertility powers attached to it. Diana was also sometimes represented as a cat. ***Ancient Greece & Rome***

~ The cat-headed goddess, Bast, was associated with fertility and childbirth. The word for cat was 'Mau', an imitation of a cat's cry and a mother syllable. ***Ancient Egypt***

~ According to ancient Indian mythology, the moon is a cat that chases the mice (stars) of night. [7]

~ The fertility god, Ai Apaec, sometimes appeared as a tomcat. ***Peru***

~ Freya, goddess of fertility, had a chariot pulled by two black cats. Farmers left out offerings for her cats to ensure their crops' fertility. ***Scandinavia***

~ A cat would be rocked in a newlywed couple's empty cradle to bless them with children. ***German Pennsylvania USA***

~ Petting a male black cat backwards foretells pregnancy. ***Holland***

~ A cat buried in a grain field will guarantee a good harvest. ***Bohemia***

~ The cat is the symbol for childbirth. ***Hindi***

~ If a woman wishes for children, she should wear an amulet depicting a mother cat with kittens. The number of kittens indicates how many children she wants to have.

~ Wearing any type of cat-shaped jewellery makes all secret wishes come true.

~ Cat shaped amulets are particularly potent for people born under the astrological signs of Capricorn and Pisces.

- **CHICKENS**

~ The Bride's grandmother holds a chick in each hand. While calling on the tribal ancestors, she stoops before her granddaughter and passes the chicks several times between her granddaughter's legs, symbolising her bringing several children into the world. ***Congo***[4]

~ Chicken blood is used to get rid of any bad luck associated with fertility. It drips onto the newlywed's legs, and the chicken is then cooked and eaten. ***Congo*** [4]

- **COWS**

~ With its plentiful milk supply, the cow became a symbol of fertility and motherhood. ***Celtic***

~ The cow is associated with the Earth mother, and the Moon's fertility cycles. ***Pagan***

~ Hathor, the Goddess of women and pregnancy, was often depicted as a cow and was said to nourish mortals with her milk. ***Ancient Egypt***

- **CRABS**

~ A pair of crab claws carried on the person or worn on a necklace, increase fertility. A crab amulet is particularly powerful for people born under the astrological sign of Cancer. *Pagan*

- **CROCODILES**

~ The crocodile was revered because of its association with Sobek (a.k.a. Sebek, Sochet) a god of fertility and rebirth, said to be the creator of the world. Known as 'Lord of the Waters', Sobek was depicted either as a crocodile-headed man or as a full crocodile, wearing a plumed headdress with a horned sun disk. He also carried a 'was' sceptre and the 'ankh' sign of life. *Ancient Egypt*

- **DEER**

~ Because of its grace, gentility, and maternal affection, the deer came to represent most of the feminine aspects including fertility.
~ Deer horns placed under the bed bring fertility.
~ The deer is associated with childbirth in Jewish and Babylonian thought, and thus for some became a conception charm.

- **DOGS**

~ Dogs were seen as healing, and their saliva was used to heal all manner of illnesses including infertility problems. *Celtic*

- **DRAGONS**

~ The dragon symbolises the male element or 'yang' and makes a good charm for male virility. *China*
~ Dragons are bad luck and are enemies of fertility. Every May 1st, two dragons screamed, causing sterility in all living creatures on the land and in the sea. The dragons had to be destroyed in order to restore Britain's fertility. *Celtic UK*

- **ELEPHANTS**

~ Elephants are fertility charms as they're associated with rain which makes the fields fertile. Furthermore, Maya, the mother of Buddha, dreamt her son entered her womb in the form of a white elephant. The white elephant is thus found within the symbol for the base chakra which is believed to govern sexual energy. *India*

- **FISH**

~ Fish are connected with fertility and pregnancy in many cultures. Because fish are associated with the water element, fish came to be associated with the Moon, the feminine aspects and fertility.
~ The fish is a symbol of the male organ and thus male virility among various peoples.
~ Eating fish in order to get pregnant is widespread.
~ An Arabic woman who has only daughters will eat fish in order to bear sons. *Palestine*
~ Ancient books of charms, potions and remedies recommend barren women

to eat fish in order to conceive. ***Jewish***
~ The childless woman should swallow a fish in which there is another fish. The symbolism of the fish within another fish, indicates the desired child in the womb. ***Moroccan Jews***
~ The husband should take a fish that has been found inside another fish, and a hare's stomach, and fry them in a pan until they become dry. Then he should grind them and mix them together and put this mixture into a glass of water. If his wife drinks this mixture, she'll conceive. ***17th & 18th Century Jewish***
~ A fish found within a fish, dried and pounded, and then taken by the wife for three nights in a little wine will cause her to conceive. ***17th C. Jewish***
~ Fold pike gall and wolf gall into purple blue woollen cloths, place them inside the woman, and let her remove them at the time of intercourse. She will soon conceive. ***Polish Jewish Belief***
~ Fish are frequently used in the Berber peoples' henna designs to boost fertility. ***Morocco***
~ An amulet shaped like a pair of fish, made of gold or mother-of-pearl will increase fertility and virility. The fish is a particularly powerful charm for those born under the astrological sign of Pisces. ***Pagan***

- **FROGS**

~ Due to their rapid reproductive ability, frogs are frequently symbols of fertility.
~ Frogs were regarded as fertility symbols because of their association with water and therefore fertility. When the Nile annually flooded, myriads of frogs appeared to enjoy the wet boggy conditions after the waters receded. This came to symbolise plentiful fertility and coming life. Heket, the Water Goddess and Goddess of fertility, was often shown as a frog or as a frog-headed woman holding the 'ankh' sign of life. Heket gave the newly-created being the breath of life before he was placed to grow within his mother's womb. ***Ancient Egypt***
~ In Peru, frogs were seen as rain callers, and frog statuettes were placed on hilltops to call down the rain and bring fertility. Frogs were also worshipped by the ancient Aztecs. The patron goddess of fertility and childbirth was often represented as a frog, and the Great Mother Goddess was often depicted as a toad in a squatting position giving birth to the world. ***Central America***
~ A frog is said to bring fertility to any house it enters. Little brass fertility frogs are widely sold to promote fertility. ***North Africa***
~ Highly decorated frogs were often votive gifts placed within pilgrimage churches, requesting fertility for the desperate pilgrims. ***Bavaria***
~ A frog amulet increases fertility and virility.

Baby Lore

 Frog Charm Symbol representing fertility. **Native American**

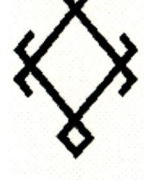 Tadpole Charm Symbol: immature frogs represent fertility and renewal. Because they change, they are considered particularly powerful. **Native American**

Frog Henna Design tattoo fertility charm. **Berber Morocco**

- **GOATS**

~ Wear or carry the symbol of the goat as an amulet to increase fertility.
~ The goat is a particularly powerful fertility charm for people born under the astrological sign of Capricorn. **Pagan**

- **HIPPOPOTAMUS**

~ In some tribes, the hippo is seen as a sign of fertility, possibly because of its swollen-looking stomach and association with water. **Africa**
~ The female hippopotamus was the manifestation of the goddess, Taweret, the benevolent hippo goddess of fertility and childbirth. **Ancient Egypt**

- **HORSES**

~ Horses symbolised fertility and were sacred to Epona, the horse deity and fertility goddess. The horse was closely associated with the fertile Sun God, who was often depicted riding on horseback. The Goddess, Rhiannon, rode a beautiful white horse, symbolic of the moon waxing and waning across the sky and of the sun's (male aspect of divinity) eternal struggle to catch the moon (the female aspect of divinity). It was a deep symbolism of ancient fertility rites. **Celtic**
~ The tribe leader mated with a horse to bring the horse's fertility to his tribe. **Celtic**
~ It's lucky to lead a horse through your house because of the horse's association with fertility and crops. **Celtic**
~ Hobbyhorses were originally part of Beltane (May Day) fertility rites. **Celtic**

~ Horseshoes and horseshoe-shaped jewellery or charms promote fertility, because of their association with horses and luck. *Pagan*
~ Ensure that a horseshoe's prongs are facing upwards; else you may have difficulties conceiving. There is the tale of how a farmer turned his down-turned horseshoe around, and his previously empty barn became full and his wife presented him with twins. *UK* [3]

- **INSECTS**

~ A piece of termite mound is said to have a close relationship to the Genie of the forest who grants fertility. Grandma applies earth from a termite mound to her granddaughter's clitoris saying, 'May the children in your womb be as numerous as termites.' *Congo* [4]
~ After a ritual washing, a healer mixes faeces and earth from a queen termite's chamber in water and gives it to the woman to drink. She says, 'Be happy, for you will give birth like a queen termite and bring joy to your home.' *Congo* [4]
~ Ladybirds grant wishes. *UK*
~ The Cricket is a fertility symbol and often one of the ways Kokopelli, the Seed Bringer God is depicted. *Native American*
~ Dragonflies are found around water and are associated with fertility and rebirth. They are also considered messengers of birth. *Native American*

- **MICE**

~ Mice are unlucky, and in legend are said to destroy fertility. Warriors disguised as mice ravaged Manawydon's wheat and destroyed the fertility of his land. *Celtic*

- **PIGS**

~ The pig's rounded shape suggests pregnancy, fertility and abundance. *Pagan*

- **RABBITS**

~ Rabbits are amazingly fertile, so it's no surprise they are regarded as fertility symbols by many cultures.
~ Rabbits are linked with the fertility goddess, Oestre. Oestre is the source of our word 'Easter'. The Easter bunny was originally a fertility symbol. *Anglo-Saxon*
~ The rabbit's foot, worn as an amulet, wards off evil, and increases luck and fertility.

- **SHEEP**

~ The God, Khnum, who created children on his potter's wheel, was depicted with a ram's head. *Ancient Egypt*
~ Use an amulet shaped like a lamb to increase female fertility. An amulet in the shape of a ram will increase male virility and is particularly potent for those born under the sign of Aries. *Pagan*
~ A ram's head on a serpent's body combines the symbolism of fertility with

the snake's association with renewal. *Celtic*

 Ram's Horn fertility charm symbol for male fertility. ***Turkey***

- **SNAKES & REPTILES**

~ Pythons are very fertile, and lay up to sixty eggs a year. A python eggshell is burnt and its ashes put into a glass of water. After some magical rites, the woman drinks the concoction, taking into herself the python's fertility. ***Congo***[4]
~ Snakes are linked with renewal and new life. ***Celtic***

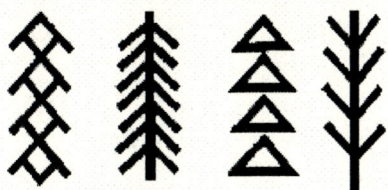 Snake Fertility Symbol. The snake is connected with the male sexual organ, and found in many fertility rituals. He is usually depicted with his tongue extended. ***Native American***

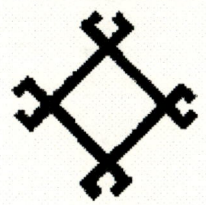 Snake and Fish Skeletons Fertility Symbol: The snake represents the phallus, fertility, and healing powers. ***Berber Morocco***

- **SPIDERS**

~ Spiders were said to have weaved a web over the Baby Jesus, and thus protected him from Herod. Therefore, it's bad luck to kill a spider as they protect children, and in some areas were thought to be a pregnancy charm. ***UK***
~ Spiderwoman is seen as The Creatrix, an extremely potent fertility symbol. ***Native American***

Spider henna tattoo fertility charm design ***Berber Morocco***

- **STORKS**

~ The stork is a fertility symbol associated with birth and spring. The idea of the Stork delivering newborn babies comes from the legend that the souls of unborn children lived in watery areas. Since storks frequently visited these areas, they were thought to have gathered the babies' souls there and then delivered them to the parents. *Europe & USA*

~ Storks were sacred to Venus, goddess of love and fertility. *Ancient Rome*

~ Storks can cause a woman to become pregnant just by looking at her. *USA*

~ To draw storks to your house, make them a nest on the chimney with your left hand. *UK & USA*

~ Seeing two storks is an omen of pregnancy. *Europe*

- **TURTLES**

Turtle Fertility Symbol: represents female power, fertility, and perseverance. *Native American*

THE PLANT KINGDOM

~ Dock seed tied to a woman's left arm will prevent her from being barren. *Ireland*[15]

~ Red clover, red raspberry leaves, primrose, dong quai root, false unicorn root and nettle leaves, all boost fertility when ingested, or hung over or under the marital bed. *Pagan*

~ Eating parsley brings fertility, and if a woman sows parsley seed, she'll soon have a child. *UK*

~ The lotus flower is widely associated with fertility. Sri-Laksmi is the Lotus Goddess with power over fertility. The base chakra, Muladhara, which governs sexual activity, has the four-leaf lotus as its symbol. The chakra is ruled by Dakini and Brahma, the supreme creative god who sat on a lotus blossom while dreaming the creation of the universe into being. *India*

~ A lotus, 'Sesen', was symbolic of the sun, creation and rebirth. The lotus was linked with the creation of man from the beginning of the world. According to one creation myth, a lotus flower emerged out of Nun, the primeval watery chaos, together with a single mound of dry land. The lotus blossoms opened, and revealed the Sun God, Atum, as a child. *Ancient Egypt*

~ A woman's uncle places squash with white shells into a ritual basket and mixes in dirt from his niece's footprints. The uncle rubs this on his niece's back and lower abdomen and gives her some to eat to make her as fertile as a squash plant. *Congo* [4]

~ A father, sensing his death is near, gives white kaolin to his children to eat to bless them with lots of children. He rubs some on their forearms to give them the encouragement they need to work hard to be able to feed these children, and spits some in the palms of their hands to give them good fortune. ***Congo*** [4]

MISTLETOE

~ Mistletoe's white berries link it to the moon, and therefore to the goddess of the moon, Diana (a.k.a. Artemis), and all her fertility aspects. Diana wore a crown of mistletoe as an emblem of fertility and immortality. ***Ancient Rome & Greece***
~ Mistletoe is associated with Frigga, the fertility goddess. ***Scandinavia***
~ Mistletoe was said to be a fertility gift from the Queen of Heaven.
~ Mistletoe is a powerful protective charm from evil spells and spirits causing infertility when worn as a ring or garland around the neck.
~ A piece of mistletoe carried about by a woman helps her conceive. ***Italy***
~ Mistletoe's tiny 'ball' like berries represent male genitalia and thus male virility.
~ Mistletoe's Druidic name signifies 'all healer.' A potion made from it caused barren animals and women to be fertile. For the Celts, mistletoe which grew upon the willow had the greatest strength as the willow tree was especially sacred.[18] In Germany, mistletoe was called 'Gut Hyl' meaning 'all heal'. One of its uses was as a fertility drug.

ROSES

~ The rose is associated with the feminine aspects including fertility. The rose's thorns are fiercely protective guarding from evil attack.
~ The Archangel Raphael, chiefly responsible for healing, is represented by a yellow rose. Visualising or using its form or symbol as a charm is said to invoke his powers.

SEEDS

~ Seeds, because of their obvious parallel with 'male seed', are particularly associated with male virility.
~ Some men wore small bags containing fertile seeds around their necks to increase their virility.
~ Growing seeds in small trays under the marital bed is said to be a kind of homeopathic magic (that is 'like attracting like,' so as the seed grows in the tray, the male seed grows in the woman's womb). ***Pagan***

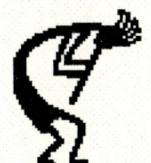

Kokopelli, 'the seed bringer and water sprinkler' is a common fertility symbol throughout the Southwest USA. He is associated with female and male fertility, and protecting seeds. Usually depicted as old and bent under his heavy load, he visits various communities, impregnating the young women drawn to his flute playing. He is sometimes featured with a large phallus. *Native American*

TREES

~ 'Touching wood' comes from the belief that each tree possessed a god's soul, and touching the wood invoked the deity to answer a specific request.
~ The ancient faith in the fertilising power of the tree spirit is shown in the once common custom of placing a green branch in the home on May Day. *Europe* [19]
~ Knocking on wood three times chases evil causing infertility away.
~ Barren Kirjiz women roll themselves on the ground under a solitary apple tree to conceive. *Turkestan*
~ Trees are worshipped, and fertility amulets are hung on trees to promote conception. *New Guinea, Iraq, Egypt & Morocco*
~ Women (and men) tie strips of cloth onto the branches of the Zarur tree, promising to untie them on conception. *Islamic* [20]
~ When a woman yearns for a baby, she takes a stone and deposits it at the foot of the Zarur tree, or fixes it somewhere between its branches. *Bedouin*
~ The Birch tree is said to 'birth things' and is used in fertility magic. *Celtic*
~ Oak trees and acorns are powerful fertility symbols. Acorns gathered at night are potent conception charms. *Celtic*
~ Wild fig is a fertility symbol. *Celtic*
~ Pine trees are powerful fertility symbols. Pine needles, cones and nuts are all used to induce conception. *Celtic*
~ A pinecone represents life, fertility, and growth. Pinecones and pine nuts should be gathered at night and then put into cloth bags to form fertility charms to be carried or put under the pillow. *Pagan*
~ An ancient gypsy belief says the first human beings were made from the leaves of trees. The following children's song demonstrates the belief:
'Our father went into a wood,
There he cut a boy,
Laid it in mother's bed,
So a boy comes.' *Transylvanian Gypsy* [7]
~ The Greeks, the Norsemen and Algonkin Indians (USA) believed that man was made from an ash tree. [7]

CHAPTER 5
FOOD & FERTILITY

~ Women get a blessed apple from a priest and pronounce over it an incantation to Santa Anna to conceive. ***Tuscany Romany Gypsy***[7]
~ Eating grapes increases fertility. Because of their seeds, grapes are particularly good for boosting male sperm count.
~ At Neith's festival, the 'great mother of all life,' oil and salt was burnt in lamps. Salt symbolised the creation of life, and the light symbolised life coming into existence out of darkness. ***Ancient Egypt***
~ Salt is good for cleansing away the power of witches or spirits that may be causing infertility. ***Jewish & Pagan***
~ Eating cabbage is said to promote childbearing, hence the myth babies are found under the cabbage patch. ***UK***
~ If children pile cabbage stalks around the doors and windows of the house on Halloween, the fairies will bring them a new brother or sister. ***Scotland***[11]
~ Eating lettuce promotes pregnancies in young women. ***UK***
~ Milk and honey as symbols of fertility appear in most of the ancient writings. ***Jewish & Babylonian***
~ The banana tree is a prolific producer, and because of this is seen as a fertility symbol in many cultures.
~ A healer mixes burnt banana ashes with spring water and other material, places this into a cone made out of banana leaves and gives it to the woman to drink. The healer prays, 'Banana tree, this woman has become yours. Make her as fertile as you are.' The healer ties a bag of the ashes around the woman's waist symbolising the granting of children to her. ***Congo***[4]
~ The new bride's father brings her into the family kitchen, places a bit of salt on a banana leaf, together with some ashes from the hearth, and mixes them together. Earth from the family kitchen represents all of the family's guardian powers joined together to share in the blessing of children that the woman will receive. He feeds the mixture to his daughter, and rubs the banana leaf on her tongue. He say, 'Go and bring lots of children into the world. Be like a banana tree. If I have been angry with you, this salt is a sign that all of that anger is now behind us.' ***Congo***[4]
~ A healer pours ritual powder on a banana leaf and adds some palm oil in order to help absorb the potion into the body. The woman crouches down and eats the mixture while the healer prays and asks the ancestors for her to become pregnant in the next month. Some of the mixture is saved to be eaten at home. The healer pours water into a pot, adds some roots and other ingredients and places the pot on the fire. The water is taken home by the

woman: to protect her fertility, she must wash her genitals with it before having sex, until she becomes pregnant. *Congo* [4]

~ Since ancient times, mandrake has been believed to have mystical powers to prevent sterility in men and animals, and to cause barren women to bear children. The Matriarch, Rachel, is said to have conceived with the help of a mandrake plant. Women either ate mandrake apples soaked in white wine or tied them to their bodies as charms. In Morocco, barren women bend over mandrake root burning on a fire, allowing the smoke to 'charm' their private parts. *Jewish* [2]

~ Mangos and mango leaves symbolise fertility. Popular paisley prints are designed with mango patterns for this reason. Mango trees are said to grow new leaves each time a son is born, so mango leaves are given to childless couples to bless them with sons. Mango leaves are also used to decorate houses for welcoming home babies. *India*

~ Mustard seed heals many diseases and promotes pregnancies. *UK*

~ Drink a pregnant sow's milk in order to conceive. *Jewish*

~ Men should eat all seed-bearing foods to increase their sperm count.

~ Because of their many seeds, tomatoes are said to bring great fertility. Eating olives and yeast also boosts fertility.

WHEAT & BARLEY

~ Wheat and Barley, along with all the grains and seed producing foods, represents fertility to many peoples the world over.

~ Eating wheat and/or barley increases a woman's fertility. *UK & USA*

~ In legend, some babies entered their mothers' wombs by being disguised as grains of wheat. The mothers had eaten this wheat and then become pregnant. *Celtic*

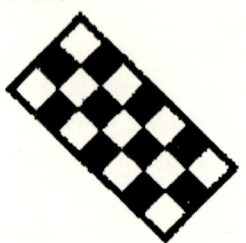

Barley fertility henna tattoo symbol *Berber Morocco*

NUTS

~ A nut contains like a seed the principle of germination and self reproduction, and so becomes symbolic of life. Nuts especially those heart shaped (*i.e.*, double), are carried as fertility amulets by Gypsies. [7] In Turkey also, a 'pregnant' almond, (a double nut) is used as a fertility charm.

~ Coconuts are fertility symbols. When a woman wishes to conceive, she should go to a priest to ask for a specially blessed coconut. *Northern India*

~ A woman can drain the superior fertility of the coconut tree into her own fertility. Women are therefore forbidden from touching the coconut tree. ***Bali***
~ Women often carried walnuts to promote fertility. In France, a bag of walnuts was hung from the kitchen ceiling beam to represent abundance and fertility.
~ A good crop of nuts is said to herald a large number of births in that district over the next year. An old saying states, 'Good nutting year; plenty of boy babies.' ***UK***

POMEGRANATES

~ Pomegranates, because of their many seeds, represent fertility in many cultures.
~ Ancient temples were decorated with highly decorated pomegranates, often at the top of pillars, to plead with the gods for fertility. ***Ancient Babylon, Israel, Asia***

EGGS

~ In many cultures, eggs symbolise fertility and birth.
~ Eggs were painted with magic symbols and cast into flames or buried as offerings to the fertility goddess. ***Pagan***
~ Coloured eggs were given as gifts during ancient spring festivals celebrating fertility. Different coloured eggs were taken from bird's nests and used to make fertility charms to be eaten. The hunt through the woods for these eggs evolved into the Easter Egg Hunt. ***Europe***
~ Eggs were painted yellow or gold and used in rituals to honour the Sun God who brought fertility.
~ Eating eggs increases fertility. The egg's fertility powers would be further increased if sun and other fertility symbols were painted upon its surface before being boiled. ***Ukraine***
~ To cure infertility, the husband takes an egg, makes a small hole in each end, and then blows the yolk and white into his wife's mouth who then swallows it. ***Romany Gypsy*** [7]
~ Finding a double yolk in an egg means someone in the immediate family is pregnant. If the woman already knows she is expecting, then it should be taken as a sign she'll have twins!
~ A woman should take an egg, pour its contents into a jug, and urinate on it. If the egg swims on the surface the next morning she is pregnant. If the yolk is separate from the white she'll have a son, if the yolk and white are mingled she'll have a daughter. ***Romany Gypsy*** [7]
~ Eating a double yolked egg brings fertility. ***Ireland***

Conception

CHAPTER 6
THE INFANT'S SEX

~ If a child learning to talk says 'father' first, the next child will be a boy; if he says 'mother' first it shall be a girl. ***Germany*** [1]

~ The Mayans determined the sex of the baby by taking the mother's age at conception and the year of conception. If both numbers are even or both are odd, then it's a girl; if one number is even and one odd, then it's a boy.

~ If the first person that a new mother sees on the way to church for the first time after giving birth is a man, she'll have a son the next time around. If she sees a woman, she'll have a girl, if she sees nobody, she'll have no more children, but if she meets two people, she'll have twins. ***Russia***

~ If a man is the first to take a light from the taper used in baptism, the couple's next child will be a boy; if a woman is the first to take a light, the next child will be a girl. ***Germany*** [1]

~ A woman should suspend a needle from some thread and have someone else hold it about an inch above her hand. If the needle swings back and forth, a girl is in her future; if it moves in a circle, her baby will be a boy.

~ If a man drinks out of a cracked glass, his wife will have nothing but girls. ***Germany*** [1]

~ If your current baby looks more like the opposite sex, then your next baby will be a member of the sex that your baby most looks like. ***China***

~ More boys are born than girls because more boys die fighting in wars. ***UK***

~ When a child is born under the waning moon, the next birth will be of the opposite sex. When a child is born under a waxing moon, the next birth will be of the same sex. ***Cornwall UK***

IF YOU WANT A BOY

- **DIET**

~ Eat tofu, mushrooms, carrots and lettuce for the seven days leading up to conception to conceive a boy. ***China***

~ Eat a high salt diet, with plenty of red meat and fizzy drinks. ***USA***

~ Eat male animal organs. ***Oriental & Jewish***

~ Drink potion made from a powdered boy's umbilical cord. ***Palestinian Jews***[2]

~ Swallow a foreskin from a newly circumcised baby boy. ***Moroccan Jewish***[2]

- **SEX**

~ The Jews believe when a woman climaxes first, the reward for her husband's consideration is a son, whereas other cultures beg to differ and claim if the man climaxes first, she'll have a boy.

~ The woman should stay lying down after sex for a while to give the slower

boy sperm a chance to get up to the egg.
~ Making love standing up, 'doggy style' or with the woman on top, yields boys.
~ If the marital bed stands with its head to the north and its feet to the south, the children conceived there will all be boys. ***Jewish, Germany, Holland & USA***
~ If the man is the one to suggest some baby-making, the baby will be a boy.
~ The woman should sleep to the left of the man.
~ Warm dad's testes up before sex for a greater likelihood of producing a boy.
~ If the woman was the more dominant partner when the baby was conceived, she'll have a boy.
~ Have sex at night to produce boys.
~ More boys are said to be conceived on the odd days of the month or when there's a quarter-moon in the sky.
~ Waiting longer after the woman's monthly cycle gives a better chance for a boy.

- **OTHER**

~ Pray for a Son until the 40th day after conception, as that's the time when Baby's sex is determined by God. ***Jewish***[2]
~ Dad should sit on the roof near the chimney for seven hours before sex. ***The Ozarks: Arkansas USA***
~ Dads should wear briefs rather than boxers.
~ The more stressed mum is, the more likely she'll have a son.
~ If a hen is set on a full moon, the hatch will be roosters, and a daughter will bear a son.
~ If the hairline of the last child at the nape of his neck is straight across, the next child will be a boy.
~ The woman's right ovary and the man's right testes are said to produce boys (and conversely, the left side girls). Therefore, stimulating the right side by massage before sex produces a boy. In 18th Century France, the father tied string around his left testicle to increase the odds of bearing a son.
~ When Mum gives birth to one girl after another, in order to have a son the next time around, she must bathe her baby girl with her husband's hat and a live rooster in the same bath water. ***Russia***
~ Visualise male sperm fertilising the egg.
~ The woman concentrating and visualising on 'male' things, such as watching a lot of football, increases the likelihood of a baby boy. ***UK***
~ A rather cruel saying is that Mum is too dominant within the relationship so therefore cannot conceive boys (I.e.: Mum and the women 'wear the trousers' and Dad is too effeminate to produce male sperm.) Mum therefore needs to become more 'wifely and submissive' to make a boy. ***UK***

IF YOU WANT A GIRL
- **DIET**

~ Eat a dairy-rich diet with lots of fish and vegetables.
~ Eat pickles, meat and fish for the seven days leading up to conception to conceive a girl. *China*
~ Magnesium-rich foods such as nuts, Soya beans and leafy green vegetables also help, as do magnesium supplements.
~ Sweets and chocolate can be indulged in guilt-free as they produce girls.

- **SEX**

~ A man's testicles should be cool before having sex to produce a daughter.
~ If the woman initiates sex, she'll get a baby girl.
~ If the father was the more dominant during sex, the baby will be a girl.
~ Afternoon sex produces more girls.
~ Have sex on the even days of the month or when the moon is full to produce a daughter.
~ If the woman gets up straight away after sex, she's more likely to conceive a girl.
~ Sex earlier in the woman's cycle is said to produce girls. *China*
~ Have frequent sex until forty-eight hours before ovulation.

- **OTHER**

~ The woman should become very girly; concentrating on and visualising female things to increase the likelihood of producing a girl. *UK*
~ The woman should sleep to the right of the man.
~ Visualise 'female sperm' fertilising the egg.
~ Should you feel you have too many sons in succession, name one Adam, and the next child will be a girl. *German Pennsylvania*
~ The left ovary and the left testes produce girls, therefore massage these before sex. The father could also tie string around his right testicle to stop boys coming forth!
~ If the woman is relaxed when she conceives, she'll have a girl.
~ Dad should wear boxer shorts.
~ If the hairline at the base of your last child's neck is a ducktail, your next baby will be a girl.
~ If you sleep with your pillow to the south a baby girl is on the way.
Germany, Jewish, UK, USA

ANCIENT CHINESE GENDER PREDICTION CHART

This is based on the Mother's age and the month of conception. This chart was found in a Royal tomb in Peking and is said to have been created by a Chinese scientist around seven hundred years ago. The accuracy of the chart is believed to be 99% accurate. Look up the mother's age in the far left column and tie this in with the lunar month of conception on the chart - the G or B will

Baby Lore

indicate Girl or Boy. (NB: the lunar month does not necessarily correspond to the months of the year. In 2004 the Chinese New Year started on the 22nd January, and this was also the first day of the first lunar month.)

Age	\multicolumn{12}{c}{Lunar Month}

Age	1	2	3	4	5	6	7	8	9	10	11	12
18	G	B	G	B	B	B	B	B	B	B	B	B
19	B	G	B	G	G	B	B	B	B	B	G	G
20	G	B	G	B	B	B	B	B	B	G	B	B
21	B	G	G	G	G	G	G	G	G	G	G	G
22	G	B	B	G	B	G	G	B	G	G	G	G
23	B	B	G	B	B	G	B	G	B	B	B	G
24	B	G	B	B	G	B	B	G	G	G	G	G
25	G	B	B	G	G	B	G	B	B	B	B	B
26	B	G	B	G	G	B	G	B	G	G	G	G
27	G	B	G	B	G	G	B	B	B	B	G	B
28	B	G	B	G	G	G	B	B	B	B	G	G
29	G	B	G	G	B	B	B	B	B	G	G	G
30	B	G	G	G	G	G	G	G	G	G	B	B

Conception

31	B	G	B	G	G	G	G	G	G	G	G	B
32	B	G	B	G	G	G	G	G	G	G	G	B
33	G	B	G	B	G	G	G	B	G	G	G	B
34	B	G	B	G	G	G	G	G	G	G	B	B
35	B	B	G	B	G	G	G	B	G	G	B	B
36	G	B	B	G	B	G	G	G	B	B	B	B
37	B	G	B	B	G	B	G	B	G	B	G	B
38	G	B	G	B	B	G	B	G	B	G	B	G
39	B	G	B	B	B	G	G	B	G	B	G	G
40	G	B	G	B	G	B	B	G	B	G	B	G
41	B	G	B	G	B	G	B	B	G	B	G	B
42	G	B	G	B	G	B	G	B	B	G	B	G
43	B	G	B	G	B	G	B	G	B	B	B	B
44	B	B	G	B	B	B	G	B	G	B	G	G
45	G	B	B	G	G	G	B	G	B	G	B	B

PART II
PREGNANCY

CHAPTER 7
EATING & DRINKING

~ Eating twin bananas growing from a single head will cause Mum to give birth to twins. ***Philippines, New Guinea & Arawak Indians Guyana*** [21]
~ If Mum eats a double grain of millet, she'll have twins. ***Guarani Indians South America***
~ Eating anything that's grown double causes twins. ***German Pennsylvania***
~ Pregnant women will make a nut tree bare if they pick nuts from it. ***Germany*** [1]
~ The pregnant woman should not pick fruit from a tree because her baby may steal the tree's spirit and cause the tree to die. ***Philippines***
~ If Mum cuts down a branch of a fruit tree, she may have a stillbirth or a deformed baby. ***Bangladesh***
~ Avoid keeping a spoon with the salt container as this causes labour difficulties. ***Indonesia***
~ Handing bread to a pregnant woman on the point of a knife or fork, results in her baby's eyes being pricked out. ***Germany*** [1]
~ Don't take food from a pregnant woman or you'll be constantly sleepy. ***Philippines***
~ Mum must not eat parsley or celery as it will cause boils or blisters on her baby.
~ If Mum spills wine over herself, Baby gets a port-wine stain birthmark. ***USA***
~ Mum should eat eggs for Baby's eyesight, fish for Baby's gracefulness, celery or parsley for Baby's brilliance, coriander to fatten Baby, and citron for a sweet smelling baby. Mustard makes a greedy, hot-headed baby. Cress and fish brine make a weak-eyed baby, alcohol a clumsy baby and clay an ugly baby. ***Jewish Talmud*** [2]
~ Eat more spinach and Baby's hair will curl. ***England***
~ The more heartburn Mum has, the more hair Baby will have. Very severe heartburn indicates unruly hair.
~ Women hope for a healthy baby by handing out puffy rice cakes resembling healthy chubby babies. ***Japan***
~ Kidney-shaped beans are particularly good for pregnant women as they resemble embryos. ***Korea***
~ Eating seaweed makes Baby's hair richer. ***Japan***
~ In beginning a loaf, a pregnant woman cuts a very small slice first, so Baby will have a pretty little mouth. ***Estonia*** [1]
~ Neither parent, when carrying a piece of cassava cake, may turn it over in

Baby Lore

the hand, or curl it up at the sides; otherwise Baby's ears will be curled over. ***Arawak Indians Guyana*** [21]
~ Mum must eat of the caudle, or her breasts will have insufficient milk for Baby. ***Germany*** [1]
~ Mum shouldn't consume high protein foods. ***India & Pakistan***
~ Mum should control intake of cereals to prevent a heavy-boned child. ***Romany Gypsy***
~ If a pregnant woman tastes out of the saucepan, her child will stammer. ***Germany*** [1]
~ 'Sharp' foods such as pineapple should be avoided as they can cause miscarriage. ***China***
~ Avoid vegetables that rodents usually eat, as if these are eaten during pregnancy, Baby will be born with a missing body part. ***Native American***
~ Sour or bitter foods cause miscarriages. ***Pacific Islands***
~ Mum should not eat anything hairy like peaches, or Baby will be hairy. ***Portugal***
~ Too many vegetables will cause Baby to have a big head (and therefore cause a difficult labour). ***Thailand***
~ Cabbage and cucumber will cause a colicky baby. ***Pacific Islands***
~ Mum must eat very little and not eat sticky food like bananas or milk that 'cling' to her uterus. ***India***
~ If Mum eats snails, Baby will be slow in learning to walk. ***Romany Gypsy*** [7]
~ If a pregnant woman stands and eats before the bread cupboard, Baby will have the 'wasting worm'. ***France*** [1]
~ Dad should avoid eating while lying down or his wife will have difficulties during labour. ***Indonesia***
~ Pregnant women should not use knives or even hold one. ***Taiwan***
~ Eating red foods such as strawberries, beets, or jam sandwiches will mark Baby with a bright red birthmark.
~ Eat foods light in colour so Baby will be light-skinned, or eat foods dark in colour so Baby will be tanned. ***Philippines***
~ Eating saffron gives Baby a good colour. ***India***
~ Apples give a child fair skin and rosy cheeks. ***Korea***

FISH & SEAFOOD
~ If mum eats fish, Baby will be slow in learning to speak. ***Romany Gypsy*** [7]
~ Mum should not eat fish. ***India & Pakistan***
~ Any white fish will cause difficulties during pregnancy. ***Pacific Islands***
~ When cleaning a fish, a pregnant woman must not cut off the fins. She must not eat fish with much blood in it. She may also only eat the tail portion of a fish. Breaking these rules will result in something being wrong with Baby. ***Guyana Indians*** [21]

Pregnancy

~ Eating crab results in a mischievous baby, and squid causes the uterus to stick during delivery. ***China***
~ Dad must not eat the Haimara lest Baby be blind (the outer coating of the fish's eye suggesting cataracts) or the labba, lest Baby's mouth protrude like the labba's, or lest Baby be spotted like the labba, the spots ultimately becoming ulcers. ***Carib & Akawai Indians Guyana*** [21]

MEAT

~ Mum or dad must not kill living things as it's bad luck. Neither should Mum look at an animal's dead body or cut any meat. ***Navajo Tribe USA***
~ Torturing, striking or killing an animal curses the baby. Anthropomorphic results may also occur, for example if a rat is struck, the newborn will either look like a rat or behave like one. ***China***
~ Mum must not slaughter an animal, as it will cause stillbirth or deformities. ***Bangladesh***
~ Too much meat will cause Baby to have a big head. ***Thailand***
~ During pregnancy, neither the woman nor her husband are permitted to eat the flesh of any pregnant animal as it's bad luck.
~ The heart, liver, and entrails of an animal may not be eaten by Mum or Dad as it causes great trouble for Baby.
~ Cooking for a man is strictly prohibited to a pregnant woman: she may however 'clean' meat, but in cleaning any animal she mustn't cut off its ears or nails. ***Guyana Indians*** [21]
~ Meat must be avoided by pregnant woman. If Mum eats any meat, any other being eating it will suffer. If a domestic animal or tame bird eats it, it will die; if a dog eats it, it will become incapable of hunting; and if a man eats it, he'll be unable to shoot that particular kind of animal anymore. Any game hunted by dogs is strictly forbidden the pregnant woman otherwise the dog is spoiled for hunting purposes, the dog recovering its powers only when the baby is born. Report is made of a woman's wages being stopped because she ate the game caught by a hunting dog and so rendered the dog useless. ***Guyana Indians*** [21]
~ Mum and Dad are forbidden from killing and eating snake during pregnancy as Baby might be like a snake, unable either to talk or walk. ***The Pomeroon Arawak Indians Guyana*** [21]
~ Expectant Fathers must not eat the acouri (or agouti) lest, like that little animal, Baby should be meagre, or the marudi bird, lest Baby be stillborn (the screeching of that bird being considered ominous of death). ***Carib & Akawai Indians Guyana*** [21]

SPICY FOOD

~ If Mum eats hot foods during pregnancy, her child will be warm-hearted. ***Portugal***

~ Eating spicy foods during pregnancy can cause Mum to bleed. ***Jewish***
~ If Mum eats spicy food, she'll have a baby with a baldhead. ***Thailand***
~ Eating hot peppers during pregnancy will cause Baby to have a large head of hair.
~ Eating spicy food leads to a hot-tempered or agitated baby. ***Pacific Islands***
~ Eating lots of chilli during pregnancy will cause rashes on the newborn's body.

DRINKS

~ If Mum is sure to put milk in her cup before pouring in her tea, she'll not have a redheaded child. ***USA***
~ Mum is banned from drinking coffee, as it causes Baby's skin to darken. ***Pakistan***
~ If Mum drinks coffee, her baby will be too bitter.
~ Hot drinks must never be taken during pregnancy. ***Romany Gypsy***
~ Drinking a lot of chocolate milk will make Baby dark-skinned. Drinking normal milk makes Baby fair-skinned. ***Trinidad***
~ Mum should not drink milk. ***Navajo Tribe USA***
~ Drinking coconut water during the latter stage of pregnancy causes Baby to be born fair of face. ***India***
~ Mum must drink a lot of coconut juice, so Baby will be born free of grease. ***Thailand***
~ If Mum drinks from a cracked cup, Baby will have a harelip. ***Iceland***
~ Fizzy drinks will give Baby hiccups or make him hyperactive. ***UK***
~ If Mum drinks boiled lotus flower, her baby will be strong and she'll have an easy delivery. ***Thailand***
~ If Mum doesn't drink enough water, Baby will be dirty.
~ Mum shouldn't drink water while standing, lest Baby get squint eyes. ***Uganda***
~ Drinking iced water results in a baby with an enlarged head. ***India***
~ Physician's encouraged drinking wine for relaxation throughout pregnancy. ***Ancient Rome***

FOOD CRAVINGS

~ If Mum craves bread crusts, she'll have a boy. If she dislikes crusts, she'll have a girl.
~ If Mum craves sweets, she'll have a girl. If she craves salty foods, she'll have a boy. ***China***
~ If Mum craves spicy foods, it's a girl, and if bland foods, it's a boy. ***Nepal***
~ If Mum craves meat, cheese, or sour foods, it's a boy.
~ Mum only craves what Baby is asking for; therefore her cravings must be indulged. ***UK***
~ Mum's cravings are her body's way of telling her she has a vitamin or

Pregnancy

mineral deficiency. *UK*
~ Mum's cravings must always be met, as refusal may lead to ear diseases in Baby. *India*
~ If Mum craves fish, her child will be born too soon, or will die soon. *Germany* [1]
~ Miscarriage, birthmarks, foetal handicap or blindness can all occur if Mum's cravings are not given into. *Jewish*
~ Mum should be immediately given any food she craves, because if she touches herself while suffering unfulfilled cravings, her baby will have a birthmark in the same spot where she touched, shaped like the desired food. In the West Indies, this mark is called a 'wish'. If the food isn't available, Mum must not touch her face or neck in an attempt to limit Baby's disfigurement.
~ Wishing for anything red to eat or drink can mark Baby with a birthmark. Mum must particularly not crave wine as Baby may get a port-wine stain birthmark.
~ Mums carrying boys will crave more carbohydrates and generally consume more calories than Mums carrying girls.
~ When eating with a pregnant woman, you must defer to her anything on the table that she may want, or you'll get a stye in your eye. *Dominican Republic*
~ Baby may be born with a fish-head if mum does not give in to her craving to eat fish. *French Canada*
~ Mint or cinnamon deals with Pica cravings. *Jewish*

CHAPTER 8
PREGNANCY DANGERS

~ A pregnant woman must not crawl through a hedge. ***Germany*** [1]
~ Mum must not crawl under barbed-wire or Baby will be born with pot marks on his face.
~ The pregnant woman should avoid all unaccustomed activity, as it negatively affects Baby. ***Navajo Tribe USA***
~ It's bad luck for a pregnant woman to hold another baby. ***China***
~ Never become a godmother while pregnant, as the godchild or foetus might die as a result. ***UK***
~ A pregnant woman should not move house or the good luck baby spirit will not move with her. ***Taiwan***
~ At a house where there is a pregnant woman, nobody may enter by the front door and pass out by the back or vice versa, as there is only one exit from the womb. Guests also must not remain only one night because any form of hurry is likely to induce miscarriage. ***Malaysia*** [22]
~ Mum rubbing her belly too often results in a spoilt and over-demanding child. ***China***
~ If a woman more than halfway through her pregnancy stands still before a cupboard, her child will be greedy. To cure it, let her put the child in the cupboard, or in a corner, and, cry as he may, make him sit there until she has done nine types of work. ***Germany*** [1]
~ Mum and Dad must avoid sex from the seventh month of pregnancy or Baby will be disrespectful towards them. ***Indonesia***
~ Mum shouldn't step over a hammock lest her child be born lazy. ***Vietnam***
~ If Mum dusts anything with her apron, Baby will be boisterous. ***Germany*** [1]
~ If Mum steals but a trifle, Baby will have a strong inclination to thieving. ***Germany*** [1]
~ Don't step over the feet of a pregnant woman, lest her children get crooked misshapen feet. ***Estonia*** [1]
~ If a pregnant woman steps on nail clippings, the impurity attached to them will cause a premature birth. ***Jewish***
~ If a pregnant woman puts her foot upon a used bark toothpick, her child is harmed. ***Zoroastrian*** [23]
~ If a pregnant woman dips her hands in dirty water, her children will have coarse hands. ***Germany*** [1]
~ Husbands must dote on their wife's every whim so her wrath doesn't cause her to miscarry. ***Doctor's Advice 17th Century UK***
~ Mocking the disabled causes Baby to be born disabled. ***Indonesia***

Pregnancy

~ Before the end of the sixth month, when the foetus acquires personality, the husband may not cut down a creeper. ***Patani Malaysia*** [22]
~ The father must not build a house when his wife is pregnant or he'll incur the wrath of the Earth Spirit. Neither must he bathe in the sea, for the seashore is thick with ghosts and this could harm Baby. ***India***
~ If a pregnant woman lifts a child from the front, either that child or her own will die. ***Germany*** [1]
~ Mum must not lie, or she'll give birth to a snake. ***Madagascar***
~ If Mum bleaches, she'll get a white baby. ***Germany*** [1]
~ It's bad luck for a pregnant woman to meet people about to set out on a trip. ***Vietnam***
~ Mum shouldn't sit on hard, rocky surfaces as it will make Baby's bottom go black. ***India***
~ Mum should be careful whom she lets touch her stomach. If a jealous person touches her stomach, they can make Baby sick or ugly. ***Japan***
~ If a pregnant woman is slapped in the face, her baby will be left with a birthmark. ***Ireland***
~ A pregnant woman should avoid contact with newborn babies, since they're regarded as recent arrivals from the spirit world. ***Ireland***
~ Mum must not sleep on her back, or Baby will make her belly burst open. ***Thailand***
~ Never name a baby still in the womb as it's tempting fate. ***Jewish***
~ Mum must not scratch the earth with her nails. ***Hindi***
~ Mum must not do much reading, as it could ruin her eyesight; perhaps even make her go blind. ***Thailand***
~ Mum sucking her thumb causes Baby to have buckteeth.
~ A pregnant woman should not sit on a water vessel, as she'll have too many daughters, or her baby will be lost in the water. ***Estonia*** [1]
~ The expectant mother greatly fears the 'qarina' (evil familiar spirits) killing her unborn child. Three months before her due date, she visits a 'sheikha' (learned woman). Many precautions must be taken to protect Baby against his qarin, or against the qarin of his mother, who is jealous of the unborn child. ***Egypt***
~ A pregnant woman must not be photographed as Baby does not yet have a soul. ***India***
~ Avoid standing at the front door in the evenings as this causes spirits to attack the foetus. ***Indonesia***

ANNOUNCING NEWS OF THE PREGNANCY

~ Don't tell anyone news of the pregnancy too soon (the general consensus is waiting until at least the 12th week) lest you jinx it. ***UK & USA***
~ Mum (and Dad) must knock on wood three times after mentioning their

good news lest evil spirits ruin things for them. ***UK & Germany***
~ You can only speak of good fortune if you first fork the 'Evil Eye'. If you don't do this, fate will turn against you for 'bragging'. ***Turkey***
~ Keep your fingers crossed. By making the Christian sign of the cross with the fingers, evil spirits are prevented from destroying your good fortune.
~ Mum should disguise her bump as long as possible so as not to attract 'the evil eye' or the attention of evil spirits who would harm her child. ***Germany***
~ Keep a pregnancy secret to avoid attracting the attention of the fairies. Fairies will harm Mum and Baby if they overhear Mum is pregnant, and will want to steal the baby away when he's born. ***Orkney Islands*** [6]

BUYING BABY ITEMS

~ Afraid of jinxing the pregnancy, tempting fate, attracting the attention of evil spirits and fairies, or incurring the 'evil eye', many parents will not buy any baby items or have a baby shower until *after* the birth.
~ Never make plans for the baby or prepare layette sets until after the birth. ***Navajo Tribe USA***
~ It was unlucky to prepare for the arrival of a new baby because this activity alerted the fairies to the woman's pregnancy. As an extra precaution, the pregnant woman was continuously guarded so the fairies couldn't abduct her. ***Orkney Islands*** [6]
~ Although baby items may be chosen and paid for before the birth, items should not be delivered until afterwards, in case a stillbirth results. ***UK***
~ A baby garment should not be given until after the baby is born in case it tempts fate. ***Philippines***
~ Giving gifts to a baby not yet born is just asking for evil spirits to make the birth go wrong. ***Russia***
~ Before the birth of a child, they prepared two sets of layettes and clothing for the baby: one for a boy and one for a girl. The linen supply was kept to the minimum as it was believed that starting under such conditions Baby would have a long life. ***Russia***

GOING OUT

~ Mum shouldn't go out, as she is at great risk of being abducted by the fairies. If she does, she should stop by a forge and blow on the bellows for safekeeping. ***Ireland***
~ Mum should not go to noisy, crowded or violent places. ***Navajo Tribe USA***
~ Mum shouldn't enter a deserted house as she may get possessed by spirits living there. ***Hindi***
~ Mum must never sit in the dark as evil spirits could cause her to miscarry. ***Philippines***
~ A pregnant woman mustn't go out after twilight as evil spirits may infest her. ***Asia***

Pregnancy

~ If Dad goes out after dark, he may not return home directly, but must first visit a neighbour's house to put any vampire following him off the scent. **Malaysia** [22]
~ Mum shouldn't set off from her house at dawn, midday, or dusk, as during these hours evil spirits become more active and could attack her. **Bangladesh**
~ If Mum passes *under* a wagon pole, Baby will be overdue. If she mounts the carriage *over* the pole or its traces, Baby entangles his limbs in the umbilical cord. **Germany** [1]
~ A pregnant women should avoid the sun as excessive heat may burn her placenta or overheat Baby. **Mexico**
~ If Mum stays out in the sun, Baby will be too dark.
~ If a pregnant woman follows a criminal going to his execution, or merely crosses the same path he's gone, Baby will be hanged one day. **Germany** [1]
~ Two pregnant women should not walk together unless one has a piece of stick in her hand, or their babies will die. **Guyana**
~ Mum must not go near trenches or sit on an anthill as she'll be attacked by the destroyer of the foetus known as 'The Son of Garbhahanta'. **Hindi**
~ Mum shouldn't go to weddings or frequent places of worship as her presence brings bad luck. **Vietnam**
~ Pregnant woman can't visit sick people as it makes Baby very sad. **Thailand**
~ Pregnant women shouldn't walk too much, or take long uncomfortable rides. **Vietnam**

MUM MUST BE VERY CAREFUL WHAT SHE LOOKS AT!

~ If a pregnant woman stares often and long at a man with curly hair, then Baby will be born with curly hair.
~ If Mum looks at a cross-eyed person, she'll make Baby cross-eyed. **Ireland**
~ Mum isn't allowed to look at deformed or disabled people, since Baby might take on their disabilities. **Romany Gypsy**
~ Admiring flowers isn't advisable because the petals resemble cleft lip and palate, and Baby could be affected by these deformities as a result. **Philippines**
~ Looking at beautiful pictures causes Baby to be born beautiful. **Indonesia**
~ A pregnant woman shouldn't watch a scary movie or Baby will be frightened. **Belize**
~ If Mum sees something frightening, she must put her hands over her navel so Baby doesn't see it.
~ If Mum is frightened during pregnancy and touches herself, Baby will have a birthmark at that same spot. Some say a child can only be 'marked' with a birthmark during the first four months of pregnancy. The Irish say if Mum becomes frightened, she should cross herself so Baby will not be marked.
~ If Mum is frightened by any animal during pregnancy, then her baby will be 'marked' by it. 'The Elephant Man' was thought to be disfigured because his

mother was frightened by an elephant at a zoo while she was carrying him. *UK*

ANIMAL & BIRD DANGERS

~ A pregnant woman shouldn't look at a snake, as it will 'mark' Baby. If a pregnant woman's shadow falls on a snake, Baby's pace is slowed.
~ If Mum is frightened by a furry animal, Baby will be born hairy all over or have a hairy birthmark.
~ Most animals, especially dead ones, should be avoided during pregnancy. *Navajo*
~ Don't look at unknown animals (particularly reptiles) since Baby might take on their undesirable characteristics. *Romany Gypsy*
~ Mum meeting a hare on the road leaves Baby with a harelip. *Ireland*
~ A toad falling on a pregnant woman will cause Baby to be sick. *India*
~ If Mum hears an owl cry, she must return the call, or else take off an item of clothing and put it on again inside-out. In Louisiana, if Mum hears an owl calling late at night, she must get up and turn her left shoe upside-down to avert disaster. *USA*
~ A pregnant woman should never pick up a cat because it will strike Baby within the womb and leave a wart or mole. In Portugal, if Mum lets a cat sit on her lap, Baby will be hairy or have a hairy birthmark. Whereas in the UK, Baby will get a birthmark in the shape of a cat, or be born with the face of a cat.
~ If a pregnant woman steps over a rope by which a mare has been tied, she'll go two months overdue. *Germany* [1]
~ Dad must not hunt or torture an animal when his wife is pregnant or Baby will resemble that animal. *Japan*
~ If Dad blinds a bird or fractures a fowl's wing, Baby may be born blind or with a deformed arm. *Malaysia* [22]
~ A man may not cut the throat of any animal nor assist in the butchering of it or his Baby will be born with a scar on his neck. *Indonesia*
~ If Dad slits a fish's mouth to remove a hook, his baby will have a harelip. *Malaysia* [22]

ECLIPSES

~ If a pregnant woman goes out during a full moon or lunar eclipse, Baby will be born with a harelip or with wolf-like features. To prevent this, a metal object like a bunch of keys is strung around Mum's waist to hang over Baby and deflect the light. *Mexico*
~ Mum must not look at a lunar or solar eclipse. *Navajo Tribe USA*
~ If Mum looks at a lunar eclipse, Baby will get a cleft lip. *Belize*
~ During a solar or lunar eclipse, Mum shouldn't move, as her every movement adversely affects Baby. She should stay in bed; even eating and drinking must wait until the eclipse is over. The belief is that during an eclipse

Pregnancy

everything takes longer to heal, bacteria are more active and blood flow increases. Therefore, if Mum gets sick or injured, she and her baby will be under a lot more danger than normal. ***India***
~ If Mum draws a line during an eclipse, its mark will appear on Baby's body. ***India***
~ Sex during the solar and lunar eclipses causes stillbirth and deformities. ***Bangladesh***
~ If Mum looks at a lunar eclipse, or touches her belly during it, Baby will get a birthmark. ***USA***
~ At the time of an eclipse when spirits prowl, the pregnant woman must hide under a kitchen shelf, armed with a wooden spoon and wearing as a helmet the rattan basket stand that is used to support the round-bottomed cooking pots. ***Malaysia*** [22]
~ In the event of an eclipse, Mum should bathe under the stairs, so she doesn't give birth to a half-black, half-white child. ***Malacca & Singapore*** [22]

FIRE

~ A pregnant woman shouldn't pass fire behind her, or Baby will be born cock-eyed. ***Guyana***
~ A woman frightened by fire has a child with red hair. If Mum puts her hand to her face, Baby will be born with a red birthmark.
~ Mum must not go too near charcoal and ashes. ***Hindi***
~ Mum shouldn't stand near a fire, since excessive heat may burn the placenta or overheat Baby. ***Mexico***
~ If Mum holds in her cigarette smoke for too long, Baby will get a birthmark.
~ Mum shouldn't start a fire, as Baby will be born with a birthmark on his face. ***China***
~ When a woman is pregnant, she shouldn't put out coals on the fire. ***Guyana***
~ Mum should be careful when lighting a fire not to throw the wood in against the branches, else she'll have a difficult labour. ***Estonia***[1]

DEATH & FUNERALS

~ Mum shouldn't go to a funeral as it will make Baby very sad (*Thailand*), traumatise Baby (*Indonesia*), cause her to miscarry (*Portugal*), or mark Baby with a birthmark.
~ A baby might be born prematurely if Mum helps out at a wake, or if she is in the room when a dead person is being put into the coffin. Mum must never remain in a house with a corpse. ***Ireland***
~ If a pregnant women look at a corpse, Baby will have no colour (*Germany* [1]) be born very white, possibly albino (*Scandinavia*), or take on some of the corpse's undesirable characteristics. (*Romany Gypsy*)
~ A pregnant woman must not grieve; neither may she look at the face of a dead person, although it is permissible for her to gaze on the body. ***Pomeroon***

Baby Lore

Arawak Indians Guyana [21]
~ Mum can't go near the sick or dying as Baby's energy is too sensitive to this. Neither should she go to a funeral or look at dead bodies of humans *or* animals. ***Native American***
~ Mum and Baby are particularly vulnerable to getting possessed. Therefore, Mum must never go to a séance, she should whistle at a hearse going past to protect herself, and while going past a cemetery she must hold her breath or she'll breathe in the spirit of someone who has recently died. ***UK***
~ Mum should not go to graveyards lest her child starve and have weak spells (*Ireland*) or she miscarry (*Portugal*). If the shadow of a cross on a grave falls on a pregnant woman, she'll miscarry. This belief was so strong that unmarried girls sometimes went to a graveyard to remove their 'shameful' circumstances (*Romany Gypsy* [7]) If Mum walks over a suicide's grave she'll have a miscarriage (*Belize*) whereas in Germany walking across *any* grave will cause Baby to die. Mum must not stand on a cross or grave in a churchyard as it will cause Baby to get clubfoot. If by accident she treads on a grave, she must instantly kneel down, say a prayer, and make the sign of the cross on the sole of her shoe three times. (*Ireland* [15])

KNOTS, TANGLES & CROSSED LIMBS

~ If a pregnant woman ties knots, braids anything or makes anything fast, Baby will be constricted in making his entrance into the world. Tying of a knot 'ties her up', obstructing and perhaps preventing the delivery, or delaying her convalescence after the birth. ***Navajo Tribe USA***
~ A ceremony is performed in the fourth or fifth month of a woman's pregnancy, and after it, her husband is forbidden to tie any fast knots and to sit with his legs crossed over each other. ***Toumbuluh Tribe: Bali*** [14]
~ Mum shouldn't braid her hair as this will cause the umbilical cord to be wrapped around Baby's neck. ***Inuit Eskimo***
~ Mum mustn't knit while pregnant, as it causes the umbilical cord to become wrapped around Baby's neck. (*Bolivia*) Neither should she wear anything around her neck for the same reason. (*Native American, Asia & Portugal*)
~ Dad may not bind up anything with a string or make anything fast during his wife's pregnancy (*The Sea Dyaks Borneo*[14]) and a carpenter mustn't drive a nail while his wife is pregnant as nailing might close her womb and result in a difficult labour *(Asia)*.
~ If a pregnant woman passes *through* the clotheslines or anything tangled, Baby will tangle himself as many times as she has passed through the line. Similarly, she may not pass under any hanging line or Baby will be hanged some day. Mum should avoid even the string on which a birdcage hangs ***Germany*** [1]
~ If Mum passes *under* a washing line, it will wind the umbilical cord about

Baby's neck or Baby will get a birthmark. ***German Pennsylvania***
~ If a pregnant woman reaches above her head, she will strangle Baby with the umbilical cord. (*Vietnam & Belize*) Some say if mum raises her arms above her head while pregnant, she can *untangle* the umbilical cord.
~ Sitting beside a pregnant woman with clasped hands, casts an evil spell over her. Crossed legs also cause much trouble. The goddess, Lucina, sat with clasped hands and crossed legs, and the baby couldn't be born until she changed her attitude. ***Ancient Rome*** [14]
~ Mum shouldn't cross her legs as it will injure Baby.
~ As the due date approaches, all knots must be loosened and items should be unlocked lest the birth entrance be obstructed.

PROTECTION FROM DANGERS DURING PREGNANCY
CHARMS & AMULETS
~ Mum must keep something metal such as a nail or a pair of scissors on her person at all times so evil can't come anywhere near her. ***Indonesia & Malaysia***
~ A shaving cut from a deer's antler pinned onto Mum's clothing wards off dangers and make Mum strong during labour. ***Portugal***
~ Mum should rub her belly often so Baby will stay in place and not be born too early. ***Hawaii***
~ Keep a continual fire burning in the house to protect a pregnant woman from spirits. ***Zoroastrian*** [23]
~ A charm to stop any type of bleeding: Say, 'Blood, thou must stop, until the Virgin Mary bring forth another son.' Repeat three times. ***German Pennsylvania*** [24]
~ German magic spell of the eleventh century to stop bleeding;
'Tumbo (i.e., dumb or stupid) sat in the hill,
With a stupid child in arms,
Dumb the hill was called,
Dumb was called the child,
The holy Tumbo
Heal this wound!' ***Germany*** [25]
~ A song to stop the flow of blood in pregnant woman:
'The stupid man went into the mountain,
The stupid man was amazed;
I adjure thee, oh womb,
Be not angry!'
This should also be written on virgin parchment, and bound with a linen cord about Mum's waist. ***Romany Gypsy*** [7]
~ 'Anzan Omamori' amulets help protect Baby in the womb, and enable a

Baby Lore

woman to have an easy pregnancy and delivery. Such shrines as Suitengu in Tokyo are particularly famous for these amulets. Some amulets are in the form of special 'obi' (sashes) that Mum wears around her belly. ***Shinto Buddhism: Japan***

~ Every Friday, Mum must bathe with limes, a fruit distasteful to devils, and drink the water that drops off the ends of her tresses. ***Malaysia***[22]

~ An amulet containing holy verses, special diagrams and/or herbal substances is worn to safeguard a pregnant woman and her child from evil spirits. ***Bangladesh***

~ Mum should tie a dried toad around her waist to protect her unborn child.

Hands, Fingers and Combs Charm Design: the hand motif protects against spells and the evil eye, while the comb protects birth and marriage. ***Kilim People Turkey***

Sa Sign: means protection. Tauret, the hippopotamus goddess of childbirth, is often shown resting her paw on it to protect her foetus. It's often used in conjunction with the ankh sign. Pregnant women also commonly wore amulets bearing Tauret's image, for protection. ***Ancient Egypt***

~ In some parts of the world, wolves were seen as protectors of pregnant women, as according to legend, Leto, the mother of Artemis and Apollo, took on a wolf's form during her last months of pregnancy to hide herself from the wrath of Hera. Wolves are also associated with Artemis (Diana), the goddess of the moon and forests, women and birth. One of her titles was 'Artemis Lykeia' (from '*lykos*' wolf) and in Attica, she was known as 'Wolf One.'

~ A shoelace was used as a protective amulet. ***English Gypsy***[7]

~ Pig's and Boar's Tusks were commonly used as protective charms for pregnant women. ***Italy, Austria & Romany Gypsy***[7]

~ Rose oil sprinkled over a baby item can be used as a pregnancy talisman. ***Pagan***

~ Mum should crawl under the belly of an elephant so Baby will be strong and be easily delivered. ***Thailand***

Pregnancy

~ Tea made from elephant dung brings good luck for mum and baby. ***Asia***
~ A nest built inside a house by a bird or wasp assures Mum of a safe delivery. ***India***
~ If a pregnant woman is the only one to hear an owl hoot outside her house at night, then Baby will be blessed. ***Wales***
~ If a pregnant woman sees a donkey, her child will be wise and well-behaved.
~ A woman bitten by a scorpion during her pregnancy immunises Baby against future scorpion bites. ***India***

PROTECTIVE GEMSTONES

~ A toadstone preserved pregnant women from demons and other dangers. It was often sold or loaned for considerable sums of money. ***Scotland***
~ Golden Amber has the folk name of 'Mother's Tears' or 'Gaia's Sweat' and protects children and mothers.
~ A 'Hajr an Naqdhaand' (stone of preservation) protects from miscarriage. ***Egypt***
~ Rose Quartz is said to have good protective and calming properties.
~ Red Stones protect pregnancies. ***Jewish***
~ Most blue stones protect against 'the evil eye'. ***Egypt***

RELIGIOUS HELP

~ The angels Michael, Gabriel, Shamriel and Raphael can be invoked to guard the baby in the womb. In Germany, these angels are known as Starbiel, Gastrakhiel and Sandalphon. ***Jewish***[2]
~ St. Elefterios is the protector of pregnant women. ***Greek Orthodox***
~ Jizo is the Buddha of great compassion and healing and the protector of children and pregnant women. He is also the consoler of troubled parents. Jizo is usually portrayed as a bald man carrying a pilgrim's staff. ***Japan*** [26]

GODS AND GODDESSES RELATED TO PREGNANCY

Bes: Dwarf God who protected unborn children and their mothers. ***Ancient Egypt***
Chang Hsien: Pregnancy god ***China***
Curitis: Promises strong, healthy children ***Ancient Rome***
Egeria: Protectress of unborn children. Egeria's Spring in the sacred grove on the Appian Road was commonly worshiped by expectant mothers. ***Ancient Rome***[16]
Fluviona: cared for Baby in the womb. ***Ancient Rome*** [16]
Isis: the protectress of motherhood ***Ancient Egypt***
Luperca: pregnancy goddess ***Ancient Rome***
Mang Chin-I: goddess of the womb ***China***
Nintur: goddess of the womb ***Babylon***
The Brothers **Picumnus** and **Pilumnus** are Protectors of pregnant women and

babies. **Intercedona** and **Deverra** are their Allies. *Ancient Rome*
Sentinus: gives sensation to the foetus *Ancient Rome*
Tauret (a.k.a. Taueret, Taweret): 'The Great One,' protective childbirth goddess. She was depicted standing upright on her hind legs with the head of a hippopotamus, the limbs of a lion, the tail of a crocodile, human breasts, and a swollen belly. This appearance was meant to frighten off evil spirits. She was often pictured holding the Sa amulet, and was accompanied by the dwarf god Bes. *Ancient Egypt*
Quiritis: Protector of Motherhood *Ancient Rome*

ROMAN CATHOLIC SAINTS

Patron Saints of Expectant Mothers & Pregnancy: Anne, Anthony of Padua, Elizabeth, Gerard Majella, Joseph, Margaret of Antioch, Raymond Nonnatus, Ulric
Patron Saints against Miscarriage Catherine of Siena, Catherine of Sweden, Eulalia
Patron Saints of Unborn Children: Gerard Majella, Joseph

Pregnancy

CHAPTER 9
HEALTH & BEAUTY

~ Mum loses one tooth per each pregnancy.
~ One clay ball is consumed each day of pregnancy to promote good health. *Native American*
~ Mum must not scratch her tummy, as she'll end up with stretch-marks. *Philippines*
~ Mum should prepare her nipples for the rigours of breastfeeding for two months before her expected delivery date. She should bathe them morning and night, painting them with an equal part mixture of eau de cologne and glycerine. If Mum has small nipples, she should pull them outwards regularly. *Edwardian UK* [27]
~ To ease fluid retention, Mum should eat grapes, asparagus and apples, and drink corn silk and dandelion tea.
~ Potatoes or horse chestnuts carried in Mum's trouser pockets are good for piles. *German Pennsylvania USA*
~ **Patron Saints of Haemorrhoids:** Fiacre

BATHING

~ Avoid cold baths, as cold water affects bones and joints, making the pelvis rigid, resulting in a longer, more difficult and painful labour. However, Varicose Veins and circulatory problems are a consequence of taking *hot* baths while pregnant. *Mexico*
~ Mum shouldn't take baths or she'll drown her baby. *Philippines*
~ Mum shouldn't take baths because germs could swim up her vagina and adversely affect baby. *USA*
~ If Mum takes a shower at night, she'll get too much amniotic fluid. If Mum washes her hair she'll get a fever and her womb will swell up. *Thailand*
~ Mum mustn't bathe in the river or go near the sea, as this is where evil spirits live. *India*

DRESS CODE

~ Baby will be depressed if Mum wears dark clothes during her pregnancy.
~ Mum shouldn't wear trousers, particularly if her baby's a girl; else her baby will be rebellious, butch and domineering.
~ Mum should never buy or borrow a maternity dress from a woman who has had a miscarriage because this will cause her to miscarry too. *USA*
~ Clothing should be loose to avoid causing Baby any mental retardation due to constricted circulation. *Portugal*
~ If Mum ties a cord round her waist, her child will be hanged. *Germany* [1]
~ Mum shouldn't wear a ring as this causes the umbilical cord to wrap around

Baby Lore

Baby's neck. ***Inuit Eskimo***
~ If Mum wears earrings from the third month of pregnancy, she'll dream of having sex with her husband. However, it will *actually* be an incubus (sexual spirit) impersonating him. ***Indonesia***
~ If Mum wears a nosegay, Baby will have fetid breath, and no sense of smell. ***Germany*** [1]
~ A pregnant woman should wear her panties inside-out to ward off evil. ***Portugal***
~ If Mum hangs her underwear outside, evil spirits will cause deformities to Baby. ***Philippines***
~ A pregnant woman should not walk around barefoot (*China & India*), and if she walks about with only one shoe on, one of her breasts will swell. (*Zanzibar*)
~ If Mum wears high heels, Baby will be cross-eyed.
~ Changing the bast-shoes once a week in the middle of pregnancy, will ease labour. ***Estonia*** [1]

HAIR
~ Mum shouldn't cut her hair as it takes energy from Baby (*UK*), or the umbilical cord will wrap around Baby's neck. (*Slavic*) Pregnant women shouldn't even brush or comb other's hair, as the hair's energy will be sucked up by the growing foetus. (*Europe*) However, Mum mustn't leave her hair dishevelled. (*Hindi*)
~ After the engagement of the midwife in the seventh month, Dad may not get his hair cut, for fear of the placenta breaking. ***Malaysia*** [22]
~ The father parts mother's hair three times upward from the front to the back, to assure the ripening of the embryo. ***Hindi***

TO MAKE AN EASIER LABOUR
~ Massage Mum's back and belly with olive oil throughout pregnancy to help the baby slide out easily when it's time.
~ Eating lots of ghee near term acts as a lubricant for Baby to slide out easily. ***India***
~ If Mum jumps over a pipe through which a bell is being cast, it will lighten her labour. ***Germany*** [1]
~ A pregnant woman is usually wished 'Kali Lefteria', which literally means, 'Good Liberation'. ***Greece***
~ Mum should not sit on any stairs as it causes a long labour. (*Asia*) Neither husband nor wife may sit at the top of the stairs, as blocking any passage prolongs delivery. (*Malaysia* [22])
~ If Mum sits with crossed legs, she will suffer much in labour. ***Bulgaria***
~ If anyone stands in a doorway when a pregnant woman is present, Baby will have difficulty coming out. ***Navajo Tribe USA***

Pregnancy

~ Mum should throw salt three times behind herself shortly before her due date to ease her labour. ***Estonia***[1]
~ Mum should pray and get a paper with five kanji on it. If torn off and swallowed in the right order, a smooth delivery is guaranteed. ***Japan***
~ For easy childbirth, red hair is sewn in a small bag and carried on the belly next to the skin during pregnancy. Red hair indicates good luck, and is called *bálá kámeskro*, or sun-hairs. ***Romany Gypsy***[7]
~ Women kneel before the Standing Stones at Inismurray, praying that they may be delivered from the perils of childbirth. ***County Sligo Ireland***[28]
~ Overindulgence in rich food may cause Baby to grow so big that Mum has a difficult labour. ***Bangladesh***
~ A child's tooth caught before it falls to the ground and set in a bracelet was considered a very beneficial charm to all women. To bear strong and healthy children, wear a necklace of bears' claws and children's teeth. ***Romany Gypsy***[7]
~ Mum should immediately turn over the tub she uses for a wash, so she'll have an easy delivery. ***Germany***[1]
~ Slivers of wood carved from Bede's Chair in St. Paul's Church in Jarrow were soaked in water, and drunk by expectant Mums hoping for an easy delivery. ***UK***
~ In the fifth month of pregnancy, a long cloth is tied around Mum's belly. It's done on a Day of the Dog, which occurs once every twelve days in a cycle of animal days, so that giving birth will be as easy as a dog's labour. ***Japan***
~ Mum shouldn't blow bubble gum bubbles or blow up a balloon as her membranes won't rupture. ***Inuit Eskimo***
~ Leto, when about to give birth to Apollo and Artemis, clasped a palm and an olive, or, according to some, two laurel trees, so she might obtain a painless delivery. ***Ancient Greece***[19]
~ In Sweden, there was a sacred tree near every farm, which nobody was allowed to touch, not even to pluck a single leaf. Pregnant women used to clasp this tree to ensure easy deliveries.[19] Women in the Congo clasped trees for the same reason. They also made themselves garments from the tree's bark to deliver them from the perils of childbirth.[19]

EXERCISE
~ Fitter women have easier and quicker labours. ***USA, Pacific Islands & Europe***
~ Dad must ensure Mum exercises regularly, as idleness during pregnancy makes for a harder longer delivery. Furthermore Mum must not lie around too much or she'll have a lazy baby. ***Navajo Tribe: USA***
~ Pregnant women struggling to walk should eat redwood sorrel. Legend has it that a tribal mother found she was able to walk the next day after eating it. ***Hupa Indians: California***[29]

~ Pregnant women should exercise daily to ensure an adequate supply of breast milk. *Edwardian UK* [27]

HERBS

NB: There are many half-baked notions put forth in this book about all manner of things, which I hope most readers will be sensible enough to just giggle at and not put into practice. Just because a whole culture believes something to be right does not make it safe. Herbs, although 'natural' can be dangerous to mother and child. All those considering taking herbal remedies *must* consult a qualified medical practitioner before taking them in any form.

HERBS SAID TO BE GOOD FOR PREGNANCY:

~ Raspberry Leaf: strengthens uterine muscles, promoting an easier delivery with less likelihood of going overdue. Increases breast milk supply, slows postpartum bleeding and helps the uterus regain tone.

~ Nettle Leaves: strengthens veins, kidneys and adrenals, and helps to increase breast milk supply.

~ Dandelion Root Tea: good diuretic that does not deplete potassium. Improves digestion, and relieves constipation. *Native American*

~ Use rock rose, 'Strength of the rock,' to give strength to the reproductive system and prevent miscarriage. Make a tea of a heaped teaspoon of the fresh or dried flowers mixed with a teaspoon of peppermint in one cup of water, and drink each night. *Romany Gypsy*

~ Blackcurrant berries are used to prevent miscarriage. The berries or leaves can be used: fresh leaves can be added to salads, dried leaves to herbal teas. *Romany Gypsy*

~ For an easy birth, mix together these powdered herbs (ideally freshly ground):
Two tbsp wild raspberry leaves, a tbsp of wild rose hips, a tbsp of elderberries or leaves, one tbsp hawthorn hips, flowers or leaves, a half tbsp of feverfew, a teaspoon dill seed, a quarter teaspoon of cloves. Pour two cups of hot water over two tablespoons of the mixture, steep for several hours, keeping tightly covered. Strain, sweeten with honey, and take a daily teaspoonful in food or tea throughout the pregnancy. *Romany Gypsy*

~ Drinking an infusion of Blue Cohosh root as a tea for several weeks prior to the due date brings a rapid delivery. *Native American*

~ To prevent miscarriage, Susruta, the father of Indian medicine, says, 'after pounding herbs and mixing them with milk, three or four drops of the juice of the Banyan tree should be inserted in the nostril of the pregnant woman. She should not spit the juice out.' *Hindi*

~ Mum should say the following to the Ceanothus integerrimus shrub, 'Deer, you do this when your young grow in your body. All day and all night you chew this brush. You drop your young without harm even in rocky places. It's

Pregnancy

your medicine that does it. By the use of your medicine it will happen the same way for me.' The tender shoots are then taken and chewed during the first three months of pregnancy to keep the foetus of moderate size. **Hupa Indians: California** [29]

~ Carrying around a packet of strawberry leaves helps ease the pains of pregnancy.

MORNING SICKNESS

~ Morning sickness is mostly the body cleansing itself, to protect the forming foetus from the toxins resulting from faulty diet, overeating or cigarette smoke. **Romany Gypsy**

~ Morning sickness indicates Mum isn't truly happy about the forthcoming birth. **UK**

~ Bad morning sickness indicates Baby will be frail and sickly when born.

~ If Mum has little or no morning sickness, she'll have a boy, and bad morning sickness means Baby will be a girl.

~ Ginger tea with a pinch of gentian, or peppermint tea with dill seed treats morning sickness. (*Romany Gypsy*) Native Americans use Raspberry Leaf Tea. Tinctures of chamomile, peppermint or fennel seed are also said to help.

MOODS

~ If Mum gets moody during pregnancy, she is more likely to have a girl. This is because all women are moody, and when carrying a girl, the baby girl's hormones make Mum even more moody.

~ A pregnant woman can have any kind of child she wants by constantly focussing on specific desired qualities.

~ Being close to water is considered good for pregnant women, bringing peace of mind and gladness of heart. **Romany Gypsy**

~ Mum's moods should be as stable as possible lest she miscarry. (*India*) A pregnant woman must observe a pure lifestyle, and read religious books which will keep her serene and help her growing baby. (*Hindi*)

~ Mum's attitude should be positive during pregnancy to keep her unborn baby positive. She should think happy thoughts to have a happy baby. (*Pacific Islands*) If Mum is impatient or irritable during her pregnancy, her baby will possess these traits (*Asia*), and if she is sad, Baby will be born a whiner. (*Indonesia*)

~ Arguments and disputes are to be avoided as Baby may be disturbed by them. Similarly, foul language may curse Baby. **China**

~ Mum must cross her fingers when around others to avoid their bad thoughts going into her and affecting Baby. **Portugal**

~ A pregnant woman must not laugh. **Pomeroon Arawak Indians Guyana** [21]

~ Mum shouldn't hold grudges while pregnant or her baby will look like the person she is angry with. **Asia**

Baby Lore

~ If Mum is jealous of someone, Baby will be born crippled. ***Pacific Islands***

~ If Mum is subject to any trauma, her baby will be marked by it in some way. The author knows of a case where a pregnant woman's cousin was seriously injured in a road accident. Consequently, he was in intensive care, and had to have a metal plate put in his head. This was all very traumatic for the family, and when the baby was born, the family weren't at all surprised to see a 'Mohawk' birthmark all the way down the baby's head, matching the exact location of the metal plate in the injured cousin's head. ***UK***

~ Cleaning the toilet gives Baby beauty. Since the toilet is looked on as the dirtiest thing in the home, the reward for humbling self and doing it joyfully is to receive beauty. ***Japan***

CHAPTER 10
OTHER PREGNANCY BELIEFS

~ Saturn rules the first month of pregnancy, Jupiter rules the second month and shapes the embryo, Mars rules the third month, the Sun rules the fourth, Venus rules the fifth, Mercury rules the sixth, the Moon gives the baby strength in the seventh month, Saturn rules the eight month (a dangerous time for Baby, as it causes weakness and death), and Jupiter rules the ninth month. *Aldabi, 14th century Philosopher* [2]

~ Babies are sometimes engaged to be married while still in the womb. ***Inuit***

~ Second babies are always easier labours.

~ If your mother had an easy pregnancy, you will, too, if she never lost weight after pregnancy, you won't be able to, either. If she got stretch marks, so will you. If she had big babies, so will you. ***USA***

~ Twins skip a generation.

~ A baby's spirit enters it early on in pregnancy. Once the spirit has entered Baby, Mum can talk to him and teach him during the rest of her pregnancy. ***Inuit Eskimo***

~ The mother must educate her baby, acting as if he was in her presence at all times, guiding and counselling him in physical, intellectual, and moral activities. ***Vietnam***

~ Childbearing is a spiritual state. A pregnant woman is said to be in a sacred state. A married mother who has a baby will never go to hell, and many sins, are forgiven the mother who has twins! ***Ireland***

~ Muslims believe, according to words spoken by their prophet Mohammed, that for the first forty days of Baby's life in the womb, Baby is just liquid form. Days forty to eighty are spent by Baby forming into a clot of blood. Days 80 to 120 are spent becoming a lump of flesh. On the 120th day, the soul is breathed into Baby. Allah then sends his Angel to Baby with instructions concerning four things. The angel writes down the child's means of livelihood, his death, his deeds, and his fortune. ***Islamic***

PREGNANCY CEREMONIES

~ In the third month of pregnancy, once conception is certain, the 'Pumsavana' ritual aims to charm the foetus into becoming a boy. The rite is performed when the moon is on a male constellation, as this is regarded as the best time for producing a boy. ***Hindi***

~ About four to five months after the first symptoms of pregnancy, Mum begins to observe certain taboos. At the same time, a long grass petticoat is made for her to wear after the birth by female relatives, who also perform magic over it to benefit Baby. Mum is then taken to the sea, where the women that made the petticoat bathe her in the salt water to make the birth easier. During the ceremonial bathing, the spirit child properly enters the womb. ***Trobriand Islanders Melanesia***[10]

~ The ceremony of 'cutting of the swaddling clothes' is held during the fifth month of pregnancy. A party is held, and the cloth to make Baby's first outfit is ceremonially cut. As the cut is made, Mum throws white sugared almonds onto the cloth to symbolise a sweet future for Baby. ***Spanish & Portuguese Jews***

~ During the seventh month of pregnancy, the 'Seemantham' ceremony is held. A prayer to fire is recited to soothe Mum, while sweet music is played to refine Baby's ears and musical taste. ***Hindi***

~ In the seventh month of a first pregnancy, a palm blossom is swathed to represent a baby. This doll, adorned with flowers, is laid on a tray and the tray placed in a cradle made of three, five or seven layers of cloth according to the rank of the parents. Midwife and magician sprinkle rice paste on doll and cradle. The midwife rocks the cradle, crooning baby songs. Then she gives the doll to Mum and Dad and all their relatives to dandle. Finally the doll is put back into the cradle and left there until the next day, when it is broken up and thrown into water. This ritual is designed to ease delivery. ***Perak Malaysia***[22]

~ In the seventh month of a first pregnancy, Mum and Dad are bathed in the river with various ritual items, while a white cloth is stretched above their heads, coconut palms are waved over them seven times, and they are drenched with charmed water to avert evil. Two candles are lit and carried thrice about their heads, and they must face the light with direct glances to avoid Baby becoming squint-eyed. Then they return to the house, where Mum lies on the floor with shawls beneath her. The midwife seizes the ends of the first shawl and rocks Mum slowly as in a hammock, removes it, seizes the ends of the next shawl and repeats the performance seven times. The midwife then empties the contents of a betel tray: if all of them drop together, it's a sign delivery will be easy. ***Malaysia***[22]

~ Mum lies down on a piece of white cloth with rice. While others watch and pray, the midwife rolls a coconut on mum's belly. Then the coconut is rolled towards the wall. When it stops, if the 'eyes' of the coconut face upwards, Baby is a boy. Later, the rice is gathered up into a bag for Mum to sprinkle into the daily cooking to ensure an easier birth. ***Malaysia***

~ The Navajo have a saying, 'whatever happens here on Earth must first be dreamed' and the ancient 'Blessingway' ceremony acts as a 'dream' of the forthcoming birth and celebrates a woman's transition into motherhood. Attended by female friends and relatives in the seventh or eight month of pregnancy, it's rather like a spiritual baby shower. After pampering Mum, dried sage is lit, then the flame burned out and the sage allowed to slowly burn

down. This is 'smudging' or cleansing the woman's home from bad energy in preparation for Baby's arrival. *Navajo Tribe USA*
~ To chase away evil spirits, an egg is rolled on mum's stomach, and then brought close to her head before being thrown away. *Malaysia*

DETERMINING BABY'S SEX

~ Mum should drink some honey in a glass of water before going to bed. In the morning, if her belly feels full on the right side, she's having a boy. If it feels heavy on the left side, she's having a girl. *Asia*
~ To get a baby boy, the husband should stick a knife under his pregnant wife's mattress. To get a girl, he should put a skillet there.
~ Betel nuts are cut into pieces and thrown like dice to foretell Baby's sex. *Malaysia* [22]
~ If Baby kicks a lot, it's a boy.
~ When a pregnant woman hears an owl, it's an omen her baby will be a girl. *France*
~ The first Christmas Eve visitor to enter the house will be of the same sex as Baby. *Czech Republic*
~ A pregnant woman tickles the spotted-back Sorukara frog to make it jump, and depending whether it lands on its back or its belly, shows the sex of Baby. *Pomeroon Arawak Indians Guyana* [21]
~ If two pregnant women sneeze together, they will have daughters; if their husbands sneeze, sons. *Estonia*[1]
~ If Mum spits on an ant and the ant lives, she's having a boy. If the ant dies, it's a girl.
~ If the father-to-be gains weight during the pregnancy, it's a boy.
~ Mum puts on more weight with a boy.
~ If Mum drops a knife, she'll have a boy; if she drops scissors, she'll have a girl. *Southern USA*
~ If Mum picks a key up by the round end, it's a boy. If she picks it up by the long end, it's a girl. Should she pick it up at the middle, twins are on the way.
~ If Mum shows her hands palms up, it's a girl; palms down, a boy.
~ If Mum walks right foot first, she'll have a boy. If she walks left foot first, she'll have a girl. *Pacific Islands*
~ If Mum likes lying on her left side then it's a boy; if she's more comfortable on her right side then it's a girl. If Mum's right side is predominantly itchy, she'll have a boy; if her left side is itchier she'll have a girl.
~ If Mum's urine is bright yellow, she's having a boy. *USA*
~ If Mum's feet are colder than before pregnancy, it's a boy, but if her feet are not colder, she's having a girl. *USA*
~ If Mum is attracted to wearing more pretty girly things than usual, she's carrying a girl; if she now prefers darker colours, she'll have a boy. *UK*

Baby Lore

~ When a pregnant woman looks back over her left shoulder when someone calls her name from behind, she's carrying a boy. ***Korea***
~ If Mum's voice gets deeper, it's a boy.
~ Drop a coin between Mum's breasts; if the coin falls to the left side, she's carrying a girl, if it falls to the right, a boy. ***Southern USA***
~ Get Mum to eat a clove of raw garlic. If the smell of garlic seeps out of her pores, it's a boy. If no garlic smell is detected, it's a girl.
~ If pre-school age boys show more interest in Mum while pregnant, it will be a girl. If they ignore her, she's carrying a boy.
~ If Baby's heart rate is 140 or more beats per minute, it's a girl. ***UK***
~ If a suspended wedding ring swings in a circle over the belly, it's a girl, and if it swings back and forth, it's a boy. If a needle on a piece of thread held over the belly moves in circles, it's a boy.
~ Scrape clean a sheep's shoulder blade, scorch it, and make a hole through its narrowest part and hang it over the front door overnight. The first non-family member to cross the threshold the next morning will be the same sex as Baby. ***Wales***
~ In Ancient Greece, if a pregnant woman's right breast was firmer, or her right eye brighter, she was having a girl. The Americans now say the opposite; if Mum's left breast is bigger than the right during pregnancy, she's having a girl. Darker nipples indicate a boy while dramatically increased breast-size indicates a girl.
~ If Mum's breadstick sinks in water she's having a girl, if it floats, she's having a boy.
~ If Mum's belly is pointed, then the child will be male, if rounded, female. (*China*) If Mum's tummy resembles a watermelon, she'll have a girl, if it resembles a basketball, she'll have a boy. (*USA*) If Mum is carrying high or out front, it's a boy, and is she's carrying low or wide, a girl. (*UK & USA*)
~ According to Pacific Islanders, if Mum looks less attractive during pregnancy, she'll have a girl as girls steal their mother's looks. The Filipinos believe the opposite; Mum appears more beautiful and feminine when Baby is a girl, and Mum appears less beautiful when Baby is a boy.
~ If Mum dreams she grows a beard, she's having a girl. If Mum dreams she eats sugar, she's having a boy. ***Jewish***
~ If Mum's legs resemble tree trunks, it's a boy. If they're trim and fit, it's a girl.
~ If Mum's skin breaks out with acne, she's sure to have a girl.
~ If Mum's hands are dry and chapped, it's a boy.
~ If Mum's nose spreads, it's a boy. ***Italy***
~ If Mum's bottom is seeing a change, it's a girl.
~ If Mum's face is rounder, it's a girl. ***Italy***

~ If Mum's hair is getting thinner and stringier, it's a girl. Shiny and full-bodied hair indicates a boy. ***Sweden***
~ If Mum gets natural red highlights, it's a girl. Lots more grey hair indicates a boy. If the maternal grandmother has grey hair, the baby is also a boy.
~ If Mum's belly gets hairy, or the hair on her legs is growing faster during pregnancy, it's a boy.

WORKING DURING PREGNANCY
~ A pregnant woman must not spin or work in a dairy. ***Wales***
~ Any activity that binds something up, nails something shut to secure it, or plugs an opening is improper activity for a pregnant women or her husband. ***Navajo Tribe***
~ A pregnant woman shouldn't do any tailoring work (*India*), use glue (*China*), weave rugs or do any pottery as it causes a difficult labour (*Navajo Tribe*), or hammer nails as it causes foetal deformity. (*China & Taiwan*)
~ If Mum works hard throughout her pregnancy, her delivery will be easy. ***Thailand***
~ If Mum begins a project such as sewing, she should finish it so her labour won't be prolonged. ***Inuit Eskimo***
~ Everything planted by a pregnant woman will grow well. ***Europe***
~ If a pregnant woman helps plant a tree and takes hold of it with both hands, the tree will bear doubly well. ***German Pennsylvania***

PART III
LABOUR & DELIVERY

CHAPTER 11
LABOUR SUPERSTITIONS

INDUCING LABOUR
NB. Some of these are dangerous practices for both Mother and Baby and should <u>never</u> be copied!

~ Vigorous exercise or a long walk will bring Baby out. Alternatively, Mum should go on a bumpy ride, have sex, take a warm bath, tweak her nipples, do several deep knee bends every few hours, and walk up and down several flights of stairs.

~ Mum should drink pepper tea *(USA)*, peanut oil in warm water *(Jewish)*, the liquid of a purple onion boiled in beer *(Guatemala)*, raspberry leaf tea *(USA)*, bitch's milk mixed with wine and honey *(Jewish)*, balsamic vinegar, mineral or castor oil *(USA)* or eat fungus ergot, cumin seed and hot spicy curries.

~ The following herbs can induce contractions: (NB: Always consult a qualified medical practitioner before taking *any* herbs) Black Cohosh, Black Walnut, Blessed Thistle, Catnip, Cat's Claw, Devil's Claw, Dong Quai, Fennel, Ginger, Ginseng, Goldenseal, Liquorice, Lobelia, Myrrh, Lavender, Parsley, Peppermint, Red Clover, Rhubarb Root, Rosemary, Thyme, White Willow, Wood Betony.

~ 'Take Parsley, bruise it, and press out the juice and put it (being so dipped) into the Mouth of the Womb, and it will presently cause the Child to come away.' ***Aristotle's Last Legacy***

~ Rub Mum's belly to induce labour. ***Hawaii***

~ Women were whipped to induce labour. If they were rich, someone else would be whipped in their place. A German Empress had twenty men whipped, two to death, in her labour room. She went into successful labour. **The Dark Ages Europe**

~ If a pregnant woman is overdue, and lets a horse eat out of her apron, she'll have an easy labour. ***Germany*** [1]

~ Making Mum sneeze violently with snuff or incense will bring Baby out.

~ Fire a shotgun, terrifying Mum and so inducing labour. ***Ethiopia***

~ A pregnant woman shall not sit down on any box that can snap to under her; else her baby will not come into the world. To remedy this, she must sit down on it again and unlock it three times. ***Germany*** [1]

BEFORE LABOUR STARTS
~ It was common for the fairies to make a mock christening when any woman was near her time, and the sex of the 'mock' child they brought with them foretold Baby's sex. Seven or eight little women came into one Mum's room at night, carrying a baby. They were followed by a little man dressed like a

minister. Finding no water in the pail, they decided they had to christen the child in the beer which the mother had brewed the day before ready for her lying-in. The 'parson' took the child in his arms, and performed a baptism, dipping Baby's head into a big tub of strong beer. They baptised the infant by the name of Joan, which made Mum know she was expecting a girl, as it proved a few days later when she actually delivered. *Celtic* [30]

~ If a doctor isn't fully paid when a woman is about to be confined she'll have a difficult labour. *German Pennsylvania*

~ Mum ties a thread around her wrist so that her soul cannot escape during labour. *Sumatra*

PREPARING THE PLACE OF BIRTH

~ A magician chooses a lucky place for the birth by dropping a chopper or axe-head and marking the place where it sticks upright in the ground. He surrounds the place with protective thorns, nets, rays' tails, bees' nests, dolls, bitter herbs and a rattan cooking pot stand, to keep the evil spirits from molesting mother and child. Thorns and rays' tails are thought to be dangerous to the trailing entrails of the vampire; bitter herbs are unpalatable to everyone; dolls may be mistaken for the baby; nets and bees' nests are puzzling to spirits because of their complexity, and a much perforated coconut is hung over the door to bewilder ghosts by the multiplicity of its entrances and exits. Over Mum's head is hung a fisherman's net and red Dracoena, whose tough vital power denotes its strong soul substance. Imitation lathe weapons are also suspended from the roof. *Malaysia* [22]

~ Mum is held in the strictest seclusion for seven weeks prior to her due date. Nobody but the midwife and female relatives are allowed to see her. On the night of birth, the door of the labour room is locked. *Russian Caucasus Jews*

~ Childbirth should not occur at the family's usual home lest the home lose its purity. *Romany Gypsy*

~ Every opening in the house is closed so that the baby's soul cannot escape when he is born. The household's animal's mouths are then tied up so they will not swallow Baby's Soul, and everyone in the house must keep their mouths shut for the same reason. *Alfoor Tribe: Celebes*

~ To have a guest giving birth in your home is bad luck. It's therefore advisable to move house quickly. *Indonesia*

~ An infant should be born in a hut separate from that inhabited by the family. If this isn't done, then the hut must be abandoned. *Inuit*

~ A mum gives birth in a miserable low hovel built of reeds, where she must remain for twenty days after birth, regardless of the season. She is considered so unclean nobody will touch her, and food is given her on sticks. *Kadiak Island off Alaska* [14]

~ When a woman feels her time approaching, she informs her husband, who quickly builds a hut for her in a lonely spot. She must live there alone, not talking with anybody except another woman. After her delivery, the medicine-man purifies her by breathing on her and laying an animal upon her. However, even this ceremony only mitigates her uncleanness to a menstruous woman's state; and for a full lunar month, Mum must live apart, observing the same rules with regard to eating and drinking as at her monthly periods. ***The Bribri Indians Costa Rica*** [14]

~ Fresh-water turtles are forbidden to be brought into the room lest they impede Baby coming out (the turtle's neck going in and out of his shell resembles Baby not coming out properly). ***Sarawak***

~ It's rare to see hospital rooms or beds numbered 4, 19, 14, or 42 because these numbers are all associated with death or pain. In the maternity section of hospital, the room numbered 43 is avoided because it literally means 'still birth'. ***Japan***

~ When Mum begins to contract, a fire is made in front of her tent to drive away evil spirits, and the fire is kept up until Baby is baptised. While women fan the flame, they murmur:

'Oh Fire, oh fire, burn! Burn!
And from the child (do) thou drive away
Drive away!
Pçuvuse and Nivashi (evil spirits)
And drive away thy smoke
(Let) good fairies come (and)
Give luck to the child,
Here it's lucky
In the world fortunate
Brooms and twigs
Arid then more twigs,
And then yet more twigs
I put to the fire.
Oh fire, oh fire burn!
The child weeps: listen!' ***Hungarian Gypsy*** [7]

~ The smallest box in the house is usually placed before the childbirth bed: if anyone sit down on it, and it snap to of itself, the woman will never have another child. ***Germany*** [1]

~ The demon, Lilith, causes great trouble for mothers and babies. However whenever any of her names are spoken, neither she nor her demons will have the power to do any evil. Some of Lilith's other names are; Abitu, Abihu, Amsarfu, Hagash, Iylu, Ores, Piratsha, Satruna, Tatrota, Thilathuy. Some people write on the walls, 'Keep away from here, Lilith'. ***Jewish***

~ The three angels, Sannui, Sansannui and Samangaluf (a.k.a. Sines, Sisinnios and Saint Senodoros in Greece) who were sent to fetch Lilith by the Red Sea forced her to swear that whenever she saw their names or images on amulets she would leave mothers and babies alone.[26] The names of the angels are often written in the four cardinal points near Mum, especially at an opening, like at a door or window. ***Jewish***

~ Put water under Mum's bed without her knowing it's there. ***Germany*** [1]

~ Thorny bushes are placed on the roof of the labour room so a dog or a cat, which bodes ill, may not cross the roof.

~ No broom should lie anywhere in the labour room because it will sweep away all the Newborn's luck.

~ A piece of iron should be placed on the bed for the protection of Mum and Baby.

~ Psalm verses such as Psalm 20: 2 are inscribed on the door, and the following invocation is recited: 'May He who harkened to thy mother, harken to thee also!' In Germany and Eastern Europe, they made a chalk-marked circle around the labour room or drew protective black circles on the wall. Other nations wrote within the circle the verse, 'My help cometh from the Lord'. ***Jewish***

~ In Poland, the Book of Raziel is laid under Mum's head, and white cloths hung at the windows and around her bed. The Star of David or the signs of the zodiac are also used as protective amulets over Mum's bed. ***Jewish***

~ A candle is kept lit to light Mum's way until she gives birth. ***Pagan***

~ Holy mustard seeds are spread at the doorsteps of the labour room. An old knife, old shoe and a broomstick are kept under the bed to ward off evil spirits. ***Bangladesh***

LABOUR OMENS

~ Some midwives won't attend a birth unless a cat is in the house; as with no cat present, Baby won't live to see his first birthday. Other midwives believe a black cat seen on the way to a birth predicts a troublesome labour. ***USA***

~ If a tawny owl is heard, the child will be a boy; if it's another, smaller owl, Baby will be a girl. ***France***

~ The owl (Kulu, the spirit of the departed) crying at night warns someone is going to die. (***West Africa***) [31]

~ The owl, called húhu, is considered the king of all witches. Whenever its cry is heard, the Vais tremble with fear as when an owl sits upon a home at least one of its inmates is sure to die.[31]

~ The Kokok or Great Owl is a bird of ill omen. It smells death in the camp, and visits the neighbourhood of a dying person, calling, 'Kokok! Kokok!' The 'Bad Spirit' also uses owls to watch for him; hence owls are birds of ill omen, and hated accordingly. When one is heard hooting, the children immediately crawl under their grass mats. ***Aborigine Australia***[19]

~ The tide coming in as labour pains start means Mum is having a boy.
~ Change of the moon starts labour. If the moon is full, it's a boy. If there's no moon in the sky, it's a girl.
~ More babies are born during full moons.
~ Baby's head sinks to the pelvis at the dark of the moon.

MIDWIVES & HELPERS

~ The midwife was reported to have many supernatural powers, including the ability to arrive in time for the birth despite a lack of transport. Midwives could also be burnt at the stake for witchcraft if the birth went wrong. *UK*
~ As soon as the Dai (untrained midwife) arrives, Mum washes her feet at the doorstep demonstrating her dependence on the Dai for a safe delivery. *Bangladesh*
~ The midwife may dress as a man to trick the evil spirits. *Malaysia* [22]
~ Never let a pregnant midwife deliver your child as her child will drain the energy from yours. *Europe*
~ A coloured midwife will 'dirty' the baby. *1950s UK*
~ The Midwife must be calm and serene so Baby is not 'marked' and will be a good, healthy baby. *USA*
~ A morally bad midwife can make Baby turn bad. *African American*
~ All women coming into a room of a labouring woman must quickly take their aprons off, and tie them round her, or they'll be barren themselves. *Germany* [1]
~ Methods of correcting Baby's position include placing a heavy stone on, or sitting on, Mum's belly. *India & Pakistan*
~ To assist with a breech delivery, two strong men are found to hold the woman upside down and shake her to encourage Baby to move. *Eastern Chad*
~ During childbirth, the womb loses heat, resulting in Mum's ovaries and genitals softening and drooping irrevocably. Traditional midwives will place themselves between the woman's legs at the moment she is giving birth, to help keep the heat in and stop this damage. *Mexico*
~ The midwife with the baby shall, soon after the birth, take the uppermost seat at the table; Baby will then be more highly esteemed. *Estonia*[1]

MIDWIFE ABDUCTION

~ Midwives are at risk of being abducted by the fairy folk. Plenty of 'true stories' abound in many cultures of midwives who were called upon by the fairies or elves to deliver their own.
~ '… a loud knocking awakened the midwife and a voice called out, 'Throw on your clothes and come with me. A woman is in need of your service!' The midwife did what she was asked, and with hesitating steps followed the lantern, which was already one street ahead of her. She couldn't see the person who was carrying it. It went through several streets, then out through the

Labour & Delivery

convent gate, and then a good way beyond the town. Finally, the light stopped moving. A hidden trapdoor opened, and many steps led underground. Trembling and praying, the midwife followed her mysterious leader, and before long, she found herself in a roomy chamber surrounded by elves, who cordially welcomed her. Before she had time to recover from her surprise, one of the little people asked her to follow him to the woman for whose sake she had been summoned. Soon afterward a tiny, cute elf came to the world.' ***Germany*** [32]

~ 'A woman, who died in 1841 at the age of 118, told how when she was a child, underground people lived in a mountain near her home town. One night an underground man knocked at their door and asked the mother to go with him as his wife was in labour. He also asked to borrow a kettle. The mother went with him and was gone the entire night. She returned the next morning and reported a little boy had been born.' ***Neu-Bukow: Germany*** [33]

~ 'A midwife was sitting at home one evening, when someone knocked on her window, shouting for her to come outside. She did, and there stood a nix, who told her to follow him. They walked to the Beck and the nix took a rod and struck the water with it. The water separated, and with dry feet, they walked to the bottom. Here, the woman helped the nix's wife deliver a child. To thank the midwife, the nixie told her that when the nix asked her how she should be paid, instead of money, she should ask for some of the sweepings. Then the midwife bathed the new baby, and while doing so she heard the nix's five other children running around and asking their father, 'Shall we pinch her? Shall we pinch her?' But the father told them not to. When the midwife was finished, the nix asked, 'What shall I pay you?' Following the wife's advice, she requested some of the sweepings from behind the door. 'God told you to say that,' said the nix, giving her what she wanted. Then he took her back home, and when she looked at the sweepings, they had turned to pure gold.' ***Westerhausen: Germany*** [34]

LABOUR PAIN

~ Women suffer pain in childbirth because of one woman, Yaburawáko. A long time ago, it was customary for a woman, when she yearned for a child, to wander about in the forest until she found one. Yaburawáko found a little child on the road and brought him home. She minded him, and he had sense enough to call her 'Mama.' However, the child grew mischievous, and vexed her. Yaburawáko said, 'You have really nothing to do with me; so why should you annoy me?' The husband remonstrated with her, 'You mustn't be angry with the child, but must mind him carefully.' She continued, however, to be cross with the boy, and finally ill-treated him. 'I'm not going to be bothered with you anymore,' she exclaimed. 'You have nothing to do with me. You aren't mine. You don't belong to me.' With this, the child disappeared, whereupon her husband said, 'Well, he's gone now, but he'll come back again, and this time enter your body, and you'll have trouble enough to get rid of him.' Sure enough, after a time the child did enter her womb, and she suffered much trouble and pain before she delivered him. Women ever since have borne children in this manner just because Yaburawáko was so unkind to the little Bush child. **Indian Tribes Guyana** [21]

~ To ease labour pain, sweet-smelling herbs are burned in a censer with which first the synagogue has been perfumed. (*Kurdistan Jews*) The Navajos burn Cedar, and in Asia, Mum squats over a steam bath full of Mugwort. The scent of amber is also said to help relieve the pains.

~ The group of herbs named after the goddess Artemis (goddess of childbirth and pregnancy), are all said to help childbirth. They are Artemisia absinthium (Wormwood), Artemisia abrotanum (Southernwood) and Artemisia vulgaris (Mugwort). **Romany Gypsy**

~ A tea made from the inner bark of the Wild Black Cherry given in the early stages of labour (*Cherokee Tribe USA*) or Cotton plant relieves labour pains. (*The Koasati Tribe USA*)

~ Powdered wolf liver eases birth pains and Ginger root compresses help ease the pain of passage.

~ Swing a hen over the woman's head to ease her pain. **Kurdistan**

~ A sharp knife or axe placed under the mother's bed with edge upward will 'cut' labour pains. **USA & UK**

~ A 'bomoh' blows on the mother's head or sprays Mum's head with betel leaf juice while chanting mantras. **Malaysia**

~ Each person Mum talks to after labour starts, prolongs the pains.

GENERAL LABOUR BELIEFS

~ Girls make harder labour than boys. **Jewish**

~ Women who die in childbirth are carried off to fairyland (*Ireland*) or become sacred trees *(Asia)*.

~ Nobody, including the pregnant women, is allowed to stand in a doorway, as it hinders and blocks Baby's entrance into the world. **Sarawak**

~ No ashes or coal should be removed from the fire after the woman of the house has gone into labour. **Ireland**

~ On the day a woman is delivered, lend nothing out of the house, lest house or Mum be bewitched. **Germany** [1]

~ A woman in her childbed has power to lay a storm from the time the labour starts until sometime after birth. She has only to go out of doors, fill her mouth with air, and come back into the house and blow it out again. **Greenland** [14]

~ Souls are said to leave the body during a caesarean section. Therefore, Mum and her family must perform a 'soul-calling' ceremony in the place where the operation occurred, to regain health and vitality for the mother. **Hmong: Asia**

~ When a woman was about to be confined, her relations assembled in the hut, and began to draw on the floor figures of different animals, rubbing each one out as soon as it was completed. This went on until the moment of birth, and the figure that then remained sketched upon the ground was called the child's second self. When the child grew old enough, he took care of the animal that represented him and his health and existence was believed to be bound up with the animal's. The death of both would occur simultaneously; when the animal died the man would die too. ***The Zapotecs Central America*** [14]

~ The Angel, Afarof, frustrates the demon Obizuth, from strangling children at birth. ***Jewish***

UNLOCKING & LOOSING

~ Loosening the hair facilitates labour. Dad should also let his hair loose. (*Navajo Tribe & Eastern Siberia*) Pregnant women loosened their hair before asking the goddess, Juno Lucina, to tenderly release Baby *(Ancient Rome*[16]*)* As soon as labour pains begin, all the female members of the house loosen their hair. (*Rumania*) In the case of hard labour, the single girls in the house should unbraid their hair and let it loose on their shoulders. (*Jewish*) Mum must never wear her hair tied back or in a plait as she goes into labour. Women must not braid their hair in the last months of pregnancy for this reason. (*Inuit*)

~ All knots in the woman's clothing are untied as a knot makes delivery difficult and painful. (*Slavic, Jewish & Lapland*)

~ All locks are unlocked to remove all birth obstructions (*Slavic, Jewish, India, UK, Holland & Germany*): a word of caution though; when the child is born, lock them all up again at once. If this isn't done, the fairies will hide in the drawers to be ready to steal Baby away. (*Ireland*[15]*)*

~ Everything around the woman in labour must be undone so as not to block the passage of the baby through the birth canal; there must be no 'closures.' When a woman can't bring forth her child, the midwife gives orders to throw all doors and windows wide open, to uncork all bottles, to remove the bungs from all casks, to loose the cows in the stall, the horses in the stable, the watchdog in his kennel, to set free sheep, fowls, ducks, and so forth. ***Chittagong: Bangladesh*** [14]

~ At a difficult birth, a search is made through the husband and wife's possessions and everything that is tied up in a bundle is untied. (*The Battaks of Sumatra*) Dad must loosen his shoes laces and untie whatever is tied in the vicinity. In the courtyard, he takes the axe out of the log in which it's stuck; he unfastens the boat if it's moored to a tree, he withdraws the cartridges from his gun and the arrows from his crossbow. (*Island of Saghalien East Siberia*[14]*)*Even swords are unsheathed and spears drawn out of their cases. (*East Indies*[14]) Dad also has to strike the projecting ends of some of the house beams to loosen them; for 'everything must be open and loose to facilitate the

delivery.' (*The Mandelings of Sumatra*[14])
~ Medicine people chant and sing unravelling songs at a troublesome birth. ***Navajo***
~ When a woman is in hard labour and can't bring forth, a magician is called in as the child is 'bound in the womb.' Mum's hands and feet are bound with a tough forest creeper. The magician takes a knife and cuts through the creeper saying, 'I cut through today thy bonds and thy child's bonds.' By releasing her limbs from the bonds, the magician simultaneously releases Baby from all impeding his delivery. After that, the magician chops up the creeper, puts the bits in a vessel of water, and bathes Mum with the water. ***The Hos Tribe West Africa*** [14]

LABOUR CHARMS & AMULETS

~ Rings are amulets against demons, witches, and ghosts. A labouring woman should never take off her wedding ring, as spirits and witches will then have power over her. ***Austrian Tyrol*** [14]
~ Amulets of the midwife goddess, Heqet, were worn to protect women in labour. Her priestesses, 'Servants of Heqet', were trained as midwives. ***Ancient Egypt***
~ If delivery is difficult, the magician lifts the end of the woman's tresses and blows down on them. ***Malaysia***[22]
~ Attending women sing the following charm:
'Seven Pçuvushe, seven Nivasi (spirits)
Come into the field,
Burn, burn, oh fire
They bite the mother's foot,
They destroy the sweet child;
Fire, fire, oh burn!
Protect the child and the mother!' ***Hungarian Gypsy*** [7]
~ In Ancient Babylon, Owl amulets protected women during childbirth and in Saxony, the sight of an Owl makes labour easier.
~ Bears are considered the helping spirits of warriors; wearing a bear claw amulet during labour will give Mum the bear's strength.
~ When the birth is very difficult, relations come to help, and someone lets an egg fall between Mum's legs while they sing:
'The egg, the egg is round,
And the belly is round,
Come child in good health
God, God calls thee!' ***Hungarian Gypsy*** [7]
~ To ease birth, Mum wraps herself in a 'mappah' or 'wimpel' (the band wound around the Torah). Additionally, a Torah scroll protects the child. ***Polish Jews***

Labour & Delivery

~ Place a tub full of warm female urine over Mum. *Inuit Eskimo*
~ Drinking water, milk or tea prevents reverse motion of the Baby during labour. *Bangladesh*
~ Strew ground black pepper under the labouring woman. *Jewish*
~ Place a ram's horn in Mum's hand, or a snake skin, or the eyes and bladder of a salt herring on Mum's heart. *Jewish*
~ Mum walked on her bare knees around a table three times, touching the four corners with her hands, to quicken the labour. *Russia*
~ If a woman's labour isn't progressing, she is made to drink a glass of water in which her mother-in-law's big toe has been dipped. *India*
~ Mix bitch's milk with water and give it to Mum to drink to aid Baby's progression *Jewish*
~ If complications arise, Mum should drink water from Mecca. *Bangladesh*
~ Eating cornmeal mush during labour helps the delivery. *Navajo Tribe*
~ Give Mum some earth from the grave of one deceased within the last forty days, mixed in a glass of water to drink. If it's not effective, the dose is repeated with earth obtained from a greater depth. *Russian Jews*
~ Wearing juniper seed beads helps labour. *Navajo Tribe*
~ Whisper in Mum's right ear: 'Get thee out! The earth demands thee!' At a hard labour three or four women pray: 'I press upon my right foot, God, the Lord, entreating, That He may deliver!' *Jewish*
~ In some ancient cultures, a linen cloth was painted with a religious verse, or the name of a deity. This cloth was then steeped in protective calming herbs such as Chamomile and laid across the womb to ensure a safe delivery.
~ The tabiz and a piece of consecrated jute or the flower of the hatisuri tree are tied around Mum's waist and/or thigh. *Bangladesh*
~ To treat convulsions, 'Black water' made from charcoal used to write quotations from the Koran, is poured down Mum's throat. *Chad*
~ Sometimes the birth attendant places a kula (a winnowing platter, used to separate the grain from the husk) below the mother's birth passage, inviting the unborn baby to come out. *Bangladesh*
~ If a pure maiden steps over a woman in labour, and in doing so drops her girdle on her, Mum will have a quick recovery. *Germany* [1]
~ In the late 1800s, a midwife customarily required a labouring woman and her husband to give the names of anyone other than their spouse with whom they had slept. It was believed if both told the truth labour would be easy. If the labour was difficult, someone must have lied. *Russia*
~ If labour is long and Baby doesn't come out, Mum must ask forgiveness from anyone she may have offended. Once she makes amends, Baby will be born. *Hawaii*

THE FATHER'S ROLE

~ A man must not make the journey to get the midwife alone, lest he be carried away by the fairies. He must pray and cross himself for protection on the trip. ***Ireland***

~ The baby will not come out if Dad isn't present. ***Philippines***

~ If labour is prolonged, the husband puts banknotes under his wife's back to be distributed to charity when Baby is born. ***Malaysia***[22]

~ On the day a child is born, the husband and wife should not say much to each other. ***German Pennsylvania***

~ Men are not allowed in the birthing room as the woman's blood is contaminating. ***Malaysia***

~ If a Cowboy father wears his boots while his baby is born, the baby will be a boy. ***USA***

~ Dad went to bed and behaved as though he were also giving birth. This was believed to ease Mum's pain. ***France***

~ The midwife attempted to put some of Mum's pain onto Dad, by placing his clothing on Mum. The ritual also aimed to help Mum receive her husband's strength. Some midwives also recited spells. (***USA***) In Germany, women were recommended to put on their husband's slippers.

~ If an unmarried woman didn't reveal the father's name, her relatives searched for a man lying ill in bed at the same time as her baby's birth. This man was automatically assumed to be the father. ***North Yorkshire UK***

~ A difficult labour is lightened by the husband striding over his wife. (***Estonia***[1]) In Sarawak, Dad walks three times over Mum's belly to try to get Baby out.

~ In a hard labour, the husband will be summoned to step to and fro across his wife or kiss her, thus condoning any sins she may have committed against him. ***Malaysia***[22]

~ If Mum had a difficult labour, her husband had to get a mouthful of water from a place where three streams converged and bring it back to her. He had to go about his task quickly and not talk to anyone on his journey. If this didn't work, the husband then gave Mum a good shaking to get Baby out. ***Russia***

~ A man should go into 'couvade' immediately on the birth of his child, (*see page 131*)

LABOUR GODS & GODDESSES

Adamanthea: (f) ***Ancient Greece***

Ajysyt: ('birth giver') Mother Goddess who provides a soul for newborns and visits every mother who worships her. ***Siberia***

Akna: Goddess of motherhood and birthing, associated with the moon. ***Aztec***

Akhushtal: (f) ***Aztec***

Angus: the god of Youth ***Celtic***

Anunitu: childbirth goddess who became the constellation Anunitu, which is now known as part of Pisces. *Ancient Babylon*
Artemis: the protector of women in childbirth and the newborn. Although the goddess of chastity, Artemis looks over childbirth because she caused her mother Leto no pain during delivery. *Ancient Greece*
Antevorta: (f) *Ancient Rome*
Asintmah: (f) *Athabascan Canada*
Averruncus: Protects infants and birthing mothers from Sylvanus. *Rome*
Bast: the cat-headed goddess associated with childbirth. *Ancient Egypt*
Bes: (m) *Ancient Egypt*
Bubastis: (f) *Ancient Egypt*
Bhavani: (f) *Hindi*
Biddy Mannion: (f) *Ireland*
Candelifera: Midwife goddess who was the spirit of the light which was placed in the room where the baby was born. This light was magically equivalent to the life of the child *Ancient Rome*[16]
Carmentis: (f) *Ancient Rome*
Cynosura: (f) *Ancient Greece*
Decima: goddess of Childbirth and Fate *Ancient Rome*
Dekla: (f) *Latvia*
Deverra: (f) *Ancient Rome*
Diana: protectress of women in childbirth and of the newborn. *Ancient Rome*
Diespiter: (m) brings forth the baby *Ancient Rome*
Egeria: (f) *Ancient Rome*
Eleithyia: (f) *Ancient Greece*
Ermutu: (f) *Ancient Egypt*
Frigga: (f) *Viking*
Hathor: (f) Creator of 'The Hathors,' being seven to nine aspects of herself as the Mother Goddess. The Hathors appeared as seven to nine young, beautiful women who danced and sang at Baby's birth and blessed him while setting his fate. *Ancient Egypt*
Haumea: (f) *Hawaii*
Heket: Midwife goddess said to be the birth goddess of all creatures. She is particularly associated with the later stages of labour as she magically hastens the birth. *Ancient Egypt*
Hera: (f) *Ancient Greece*
Ilithyia; (f) frees Baby from the womb. *Ancient Greece*
Intercidona: (f) *Ancient Rome*
Ixazalvoh: (meaning 'water') goddess of female sexuality and childbirth *Mayan*
Ixchel: (meaning 'rainbow') (f) *Mayan*

Juno Lucina: Another face of Juno, Juno Lucina had two roles. She protected pregnant woman and brought the child into the light. *Ancient Rome*
Juno Sospita: (f) presided over labour and delivery. *Ancient Rome*
Kapo: (f) *Hawaiian*
Kwan Yin: (also known as Kwannon): 'The Great Mother' sometimes depicted holding a child. *China*
Ishtar: (f) *Ancient Babylon*
Isis: (f) *Ancient Egypt*
Laima: (f) *Lithuania*
Maia: (f) *Ancient Rome*
Mabb: (f) *Welsh*
Mami: (f) *Sumerian*
Mater Matuta: (f) commonly invoked by the expectant mum. *Ancient Rome*
Meshkent: (f) married to Shai, the protector of the newborn's destiny. Egyptian women traditionally gave birth squatting over a brick, so she was represented as a tile or a brick with a woman's head. *Ancient Egypt*
Meskhoni: (f) *Ancient Egypt*
Metztli: (f) Goddess of the moon, love, marriage, and childbirth. *Aztec*
Mylitta: (f) *Ancient Babylon*
Nascio: (f) *Ancient Rome*
Natio: aids labour *Ancient Rome*
Nekhbet: (f) *Ancient Egypt*
Ninmah: (f) *Chaldean*
Nintur: (a.k.a. Ninhursaga) 'Lady Who Gives Form'. The Mother Goddess represented holding a midwife's bucket of water. *Sumeria*
Nona: (meaning 'ninth') goddess who determined the proper date of birth. Nona was called upon in the ninth month when the child was due to be born. *Ancient Rome*
Nukua: (f) *China*
Numeria: (f) *Ancient Rome*
Opigena: aids labour *Ancient Rome*
Partula: Presided over delivery and post delivery *Ancient Rome*
Pi-Hsia Yuan-Chin: 'the Princess of Streaked Clouds'. Midwife goddess who protects mother and baby during delivery. She also brings health and good fortune to the newborn. *China*
Porrima: Midwife goddess for babies born normally. *Ancient Rome*
Postverta: Midwife goddess for breech babies *Ancient Rome*
Pukkeenegak: (f) *Eskimo*
Purandhi: (f) *Hindu*
Rhea: (f) *Ancient Greece*
Sar-Akka: (f) *Sweden*

Serket: the scorpion-headed goddess assists during labour and protects the pregnant woman. *Ancient Egypt*
Shai: the god who protected children's destiny. *Ancient Egypt*
Shashti: (f) *Hindi*
Taueret: Protective hippopotamus goddess of childbirth, who scared away any demons attacking the newborn. *Ancient Egypt*
Tlazolteotl: (f) protectress *Mayan*
Thalna: (f) *Ancient Rome*
Uks-Akka: (f) *Sweden*
Uni: (f) *Etruscan*
Umaj: (f) *Yakut*

ROMAN CATHOLIC SAINTS RELATED TO LABOUR & DELIVERY

~ The Holy Mother Mary is said to come in spirit to every woman who is in labour.
Patron Saint of Women in Labour: Anne (grandmother of Jesus and mother of Mary), Erasmus, John of Bridlington, Margaret of Antioch, Margaret of Fontana, Mary of Oignies
Patron Saint of Birth Pains: Erasmus
Patron Saint against Pain: Madron
Patron Saint of relief from Birth Complications: Ulric (pregnant women who drank from his chalice had easy deliveries)
Patron Saint of Childbirth: Erasmus, Gerard Majella, Leonard of Noblac, Lutgardis, Margaret of Antioch, Mary Blessed Virgin, Raymond Nonnatus ~ born in 1204 and delivered by Cesarean section, became a patron saint of childbirth.
Patron Saints of Convulsions: John the Baptist, Willibrord
Patron Saints of Midwives: Brigid of Ireland, Cosmas, Damian, Dorothy of Caesarea, Drogo, Margaret of Cortona, Raymund Nonnatus
Patron Saint of Obstetricians: Raymond Nonnatus
Patron Saint of Doctors; Cosmas, Damian, Luke the Apostle, Pantaleon, Raphael the Archangel

Chapter 12
Post Delivery Beliefs

POST DELIVERY CARE

~ The first medicine which a woman receives following childbirth should be taken from her husband's spoon; it will thus be more effective. ***Germany*** [1]

~ Powdered neem and jute leaves mixed with honey and ghee help dry the fallopian tube, and prevent swelling, cervical pain, anorexia, indigestion and dizziness. ***Bangladesh***

~ Women should drink a Milkweed tea immediately after childbirth. ***Navajo***

~ A hole is made in the ground, where twelve types of spices are put and a fire is lit. When the flames come up, Mum squats over the hole. This heat helps her uterus to retract and heals the raw flesh of the womb. ***Bangladesh***

~ Massaging the scalp with warm oil smoked with freshly ground garlic and ginger protects against burning skull. A paste of chalta leaves massaged onto Mum's scalp prevents postnatal diarrhoea. Warm pigeon blood massaged onto the scalp immediately after delivery prevents eclampsia. ***Bangladesh***

~ To stop postpartum bleeding, Black Western Chokecherry juice (*Arikara Tribe USA*), a buckwheat plant infusion (*Hopi Tribe USA*)) or a drink of brick dissolved in water is given. (*India & Pakistan*)

~ The Omaha Tribe in the USA apply the liquid of boiled smooth upland sumac fruits as an external wash to stop bleeding. However, in Bangladesh they believe the more excessive the bleeding is, the quicker Mum's recovery. A hot compress helps to discharge the polluted blood out of the body.

~ A woman must sit up for at least twenty-four hours post labour. ***Sarawak***

~ When Baby is born, Mum should take three bites of an onion, be lifted and set down three times in the stool, draw her thumbs in, and blow three times into each fist. ***Germany*** [1]

~ Mum is given a root to eat to eliminate bad air, and a cigar to smoke. ***Philippines***

~ When the after-pains begin, some of the gypsy tribes in the Siebenburgen smoke the sufferer with decayed willow-wood while singing:

'Fast and fast the smoke flies,
And flies, the moon flies,
When they find (themselves)
Health (yet) will come to thee,
When the smoke no (longer) flies
Thou wilt feel pain no more!' ***Transylvanian Gypsy*** [7]

DELIVERING THE AFTERBIRTH/PLACENTA

~ If the midwife cuts the umbilical cord before the placenta is delivered, she

ties it to Mum's leg with a strong piece of string, using many knots to keep the placenta from rising into Mum's throat and choking her. ***Guatemala***
~ If the afterbirth will not follow, cut a portion of the umbilical cord from Baby and tie it to Mum's thigh as a kind of sympathetic attraction. (*Malaysia*[22]) Alternately, put salt on Mum's tongue (*Peru*), push garlic paste or a tuft of hair dipped into kerosene oil down Mum's throat to make her vomit (*Bangladesh*), throw a fishing net over Mum (*Hawaii*), apply pressure upon her abdomen with knees or a wooden stool, or roast flower petals in a frying pan. (*Bangladesh*) Native Americans give Mum a tea made from the whole Broom Snakeweed plant or the boiled roots of American Liquorice.

DISPOSAL OF THE AFTERBIRTH

~ Mum should not smell the blood from Baby's afterbirth for too long. ***Navajo***
~ Eating the placenta is lucky and celebrates the birth. The placenta is rich in nutrients and is said to relieve postnatal depression. (*Asia*) Tarong mothers are given tea made from the charred placenta. (*Philippines*) A nursing mother should make a broth from the placenta and drink it to improve her breast milk. (*China*)
~ A piece of the afterbirth should be kept to ensure Baby a healthy and prosperous life. ***France***
~ A barren woman should sit on a placenta so she may conceive. ***Jewish***
~ Hang the placenta on a tree so Baby will become a good tree climber, put it in water so he will be a good swimmer, or wrap and bury the placenta with pages from a book to produce an intelligent child. ***Philippines***
~ Bury the placenta at the backdoor of the house so Baby will never want (*Indonesia*) or a girl's placenta under the hearth so she'll always be home-loving and not be morally corrupt. (*Palestine*)
~ For Baby to follow traditional ways, bury a cultural symbol with the placenta as a kind of 'heritage insurance'. Buried within the sacred Four Corners of the tribe's reservation, the placenta acts as a 'hold' on the child to stay with his ancestral land and people. ***Navajo***
~ To bring Baby future fertility, bury the placenta under a fruit tree for a girl, and a nut tree for a boy. (*Pagan*) In Mecklenburg, Germany, the placenta is thrown at the foot of a young tree, and the child is believed to then grow with the tree. [14]
~ The placenta was buried near the threshold of a home to protect the house and family from fire or other disasters. ***England***
~ The placenta can be used by witches or evil spirits to cause harm to Baby, therefore it must be disposed of carefully.
~ As the placenta has its own spirit, Dad must wash and then bury it in a secret shady place. If this isn't done correctly, Mum or baby may become sick and die. ***Bolivia***

~ The placenta is put in a banana leaf or an earthen pot and buried deep in the ground so no animal or evil spirit can reach it. If anything reaches the placenta, it may cause Mum's milk to dry up, or inflict diarrhoea on the baby or even death. ***Bangladesh***

~ The Hmong word for placenta can be translated as 'jacket' as the placenta is considered an individual's first and finest clothing. The Hmong people bury the placenta, and believe after death, the soul retraces all the steps taken in life until it finally reaches the burial place of its 'placenta jacket'. ***Hmong: Asia***

~ The link between the mother, baby and afterbirth is considered very strong during the first forty days following birth. The placenta is washed thoroughly, placed in a pot with salt and spices, and kept near Mum. Considered the baby's dead twin, Mum and Baby's health is affected by the placenta's condition. Should Mum or Baby be sick, the *real* reason is thought to be due to inadequate treatment of the placenta, and additional salt and spices must be added to the pot to remedy the situation. After forty days, the 'twin' is buried in the ground. ***Malaysia & Indonesia***

~ The placenta is treated as the dead twin of the live child and is given full burial rites. ***The Ibo People of Nigeria & Ghana***

~ Among the natives on the Pennefather River in Queensland, it's believed a part of the child's spirit stays in the afterbirth. The grandmother buries the placenta in the sand, marking the spot by twigs which she sticks in the ground in a circle, tying their tops together so that the structure resembles a cone. When Anjea, the being who causes conception in women by putting mud babies into their wombs, comes along and sees the place, he takes away the placenta's spirit to one of his haunts, such as a tree, a hole in a rock, or a lagoon where it may remain for years. But sometime or other he will put the spirit again into a baby, and it will be born once more into the world. ***Aborigine***[14]

~ The placenta passes for Baby's younger brother or sister, the sex being determined by the sex of the child, and it is buried under the house. It is bound up with Baby's welfare, and believed to be the seat of the transferable soul. Of a person's two souls, it is the true soul that lives with the placenta under the house and conceives children. ***The Bataks: Sumatra***[14]

~ Every person is born with a double, and this double is the afterbirth which is regarded as a second child. Mum buries the afterbirth at the root of a plantain tree, which becomes sacred until the fruit has ripened. The fruit is plucked and eaten at a sacred family feast. ***The Baganda: Uganda***[14]

THE UMBILICAL CORD

~ Cutting the cord with a flute will ensure Baby has a pleasant voice. ***Sumatra***

~ The midwife can't cut the umbilical cord until a 'bomoh' sprays the newborn with betel leaf juice to protect him against evil spirits. ***Malaysia***

~ Putting cow dung on the cord was thought to be a good dressing to stop bleeding. It was a dangerous practice though as it often caused tetanus. ***USA***
~ The midwife gives the dried cord to Dad with strict instructions to preserve it carefully, for as long as it's kept, Baby will thrive and be free from sickness. ***Berlin***[14]
~ If the cord is kept in a jar, Baby will have a long life. ***Thailand***
~ In many tribes, the cord is placed in a medicine bag, which the individual carries for life. ***Native American***
~ The cord was preserved with the greatest care, and given to the child to suck whenever he fell ill. ***The Incas: Peru*** [14]
~ Save the umbilical cord for luck. ***German Jews & USA***
~ Burn the umbilical cord when it falls off or the child will be hyperactive and always running around. ***Portugal***
~ Burning the cord ensures Baby can live without his mother if necessary. ***Africa***
~ When Baby's cord falls off, it must be destroyed by burying or burning so he doesn't get ill. ***Hawaii***
~ Wrapping the cord in a cloth and burying it deep in the ground keeps evil people and spirits casting spells on it to harm Mum and Baby. ***Portugal & Spain***
~ Don't throw the cord into water or fire, as the child will be drowned or burned. ***Beauce & Perche: Northern France*** [14]
~ When the cord falls off, a poultice is applied and mixed with pepper to make Baby brave. ***Malaysia*** [22]
~ Wherever the cord is thrown, causes Baby to choose the profession exercised in that place. If possible, throw the cord high up onto the premises' roof for career advancement. (*Turkey*) The cord buried under an anthill ensures an industrious, hard worker. (*Native American*)
~ The cord is placed in a shell and then disposed of in a way that best fits the career which the parents have chosen for Baby; for example, if they wish to make him a good climber, they will hang the cord on a tree. ***Ponape: Caroline Islands***[14]
~ Certain tribes believe a man swims well or badly, according to whether his mother threw his cord into water or not. ***Western Australia***[14]
~ Parts of the cord are strategically placed around the camp, to help Baby become a good weaver, equestrian, or sheepherder. Alternately, the cord is buried near the house so the child will always return home and help his mother. ***Navajo Tribe***
~ A boy's cord was given for soldiers to bury on a battlefield so the boy might acquire a passion for war. A girl's cord was buried beside the domestic hearth to inspire her with a love of home and taste for cooking and baking. ***Mexico***[14]

~ A girl's cord is buried under a corn mortar so she grows up to be a good baker; but the boy's cord is hung up on a tree in the woods so he may be a good hunter. ***The Cherokee Tribe USA***[14]

~ If the severed cords of a woman's successive children are preserved together, these children will not quarrel or be disunited when they grow up. ***Negri Sembilan Malaysia***[22]

~ The cord was buried in a sacred place and a young sapling planted over it. As the tree grew, it was a sign of life for the child; if it flourished, the child would prosper; if it withered and died, the parents assumed the worst for their little one. ***Maori***[14]

~ A boy's cord is planted with a coconut or the slip of a breadfruit tree, and his life becomes intimately connected with the tree's. ***Fiji***[14]

~ Three days after birth, the placenta and cord are buried in the ground and a young tree is planted in that spot. The tree becomes Baby's tree and is called the 'navel string tree'. ***Jamaica***

~ The cord is regarded as the brother or sister of the child, according to the sex of the infant. They put it in a pot with ashes, and set it in the branches of a tree, so it may keep a watchful eye on the fortunes of its comrade. ***The Kei Islands Indonesia***[14]

~ The cord is kept for a while wrapt up in a piece of old linen, and then cut or pricked to pieces depending on whether the child is a boy or a girl, so he or she may be a skilful workman or seamstress. ***Rhenish Bavaria***[14]

~ The charred umbilical cord, put it in a drink of an alcoholic without their knowledge, stops them from drinking. ***Spain***

~ A piece of a boy's cord was kept and knotted. When the child reached seven years old he had to untie the knot to prove he was 'normal' and had reached the age of reason. ***France***

~ When their cord is handed to a child in their teens, should the girl sew it up, she'll become a seamstress; if a boy cuts it into bits, he'll be a woodchopper. ***German Pennsylvania: USA***

Chapter 13
Birth Omens

BIRTH CIRCUMSTANCES

~ A child will become great and popular if born with the umbilical cord around his neck. *German Pennsylvania USA*

~ Sons born after their father's deaths have the power of blowing away skin that grows over the eyes for three Fridays running. He also has power over fevers. *Germany* [1]

~ The child whose birth causes his mother's death is born under happy auspices. *Ancient Rome* [16]

~ If a child is born during a thunderstorm, he'll be killed by lightning. *German Pennsylvania USA*

~ A raven or Cornish Chough is a good sign as it's the spirit of King Arthur reincarnated. However, if it croaks over the house it bodes evil. *Cornwall* [12]

~ If an Owl hoots as a child is born, Baby will have an unhappy life. *Germany*

~ Children born with their face down and their arms crossed are gifted with second sight. *UK*

- **BREECH BABIES**

~ Children born feet first are unlucky (*Ancient Rome*[16]), are often spoken of as bad (*Surinam*[35]), are destined to become crippled in an accident unless their legs are rubbed with bay leaves (*UK*), and are gifted with second sight and/or have magical or healing powers (*UK*)

~ A breech baby should immediately be put to death or the entire family will be killed by a fiery devil. (*Brazilian Indians*) In Nigeria, breech babies were destroyed, believed to be incarnations of evil spirits.[36]

~ If someone has a crook in his back, he should sit near the threshold of one who has a breech baby. That Mum or Dad should stand on the inner side of the threshold and give a kick to the sufferer, who will then be healed. *UK*

- **BABIES BORN BY CAESAREAN SECTION**

~ Caesarean babies are always more beautiful as adults, are lazy as they couldn't be bothered to make their way out, will have fewer struggles in life, or are special and destined for greatness like their namesake Caesar.

- **EARLY & PREMATURE BABIES**

~ Early babies had to be born under a certain star or sun sign. Alternately, Mum lied about Baby's true paternity.

~ Early babies are inpatient and ambitious.

~ Slightly earlier babes will be fitter, more energetic and independent, and sleep less.

~ A baby born at seven months gestation has a greater chance of making it than one born at eight months. *Jewish* [2]

- **LATE BABIES**

~ Late babes were waiting for the stars to be right for their birth. Alternately, Mum lied about Baby's true paternity.

~ Late babes are lazy and can't be bothered, will sleep better and longer (as lazier), are depressives and don't want to be born, will be less fit, are clingier to mum and are more selfish (draining mum of more energy during pregnancy). They're also less holy.

- **QUICK & SLOW LABOURS**

~ Quick babies resulting in an easy labour will be easy-tempered and non-demanding. However, they're always in a hurry and are rash and flighty.

~ Babies that have been born causing less pain to their mothers are especially blessed, and are born of holier mothers. *Jewish*

~ Long labour means a stubborn baby, a slow methodical worker, albeit patient, and steadfast.

- **PLACE OF BIRTH**

~ A child born in the fields will be brave; on a bale of straw, rich; on a bundle of firewood, poor but healthy; by the mill, fragile and intelligent; and by the stove will like his food. *France*

~ A baby born near water will be calm and spiritual. *Romany Gypsy*

~ Babies born en-route to the hospital will be nomads, never living in one place for too long. *UK*

- **BIRTH SEQUENCE**

~ The seventh son of a seventh son has power over all diseases, curing them by laying on his hands. *UK & Europe*

~ The seventh son is a lucky man, for healing, planting, or doing anything. However, when seven girls running are born of one marriage, one is a werewolf. *Germany* [1]

~ The seventh or twelfth child is exceptionally gifted. *Romany Gypsy* [7]

~ The Krstnik is the youngest of twelve brothers, all sons of the same father. These 'twelvers' are the great protectors of the world from witchcraft. But they're in great danger on Saint John's Eve, for witches have the most power then, and attack the Krstniki with sticks, stakes, or stumps of saplings. Therefore, in the autumn they carefully remove all the wood from the ground. *Croatian Gypsy* [7]

~ A child of the other sex born after three consecutive children of one sex is unlucky and called 'Trikhal.' The girl is unlucky for the father and the boy for the mother. To ward off the evil associated with a Trikhal, the newborn is made to pass through a hole in a sieve, which is specially torn for this purpose. Alternatively, earth is dug up from under the threshold and Baby is made to pass under it. *Hindi*

~ Daughters should be born in odd number in the sequence of birth i.e. first,

third, and fifth children should be girls. ***India***
~ A fourth born girl ruins the house.
A fifth born girl will bring gold to the house. However, a fifth born boy will squander away all the wealth.
A sixth born girl brings either prosperity or poverty.
A seventh born girl will bring poverty to the family; she cannot be successful even as a beggar.
An eighth born girl destroys everything.
A tenth born girl makes wealth fly away like cotton.
In view of these beliefs, contracting parties to a marriage make enquires about the number of the birth of the Bride or Groom. ***India***

- **MULTIPLE BIRTHS**

~ Many cultures believe twins have mystical powers. Twins are objects of worship, can divine events, predict the sex of an unborn child, are immune from the poisons of serpents and scorpions, can control the weather and give soldiers immortality in battle. The parents of twins are also somehow blessed by default with these special powers.

~ Twins control the weather; therefore the Tsimshian Indians pray to wind and rain saying, 'Calm down, breath of the twins.' ***British Columbia***[14]

~ In their childhood, twins can summon any wind by motions of their hands, and make fair or foul weather. They can also cure diseases by swinging a large wooden rattle. ***Kwatiutl Indians: British Columbia***[14]

~ The Shuswap Indians like the Thompson Indians, associate twins with the grizzly bear, for they call them 'young grizzly bears.' According to them, twins are endowed with supernatural powers. In particular they can make good or bad weather. They produce rain by spilling water from a basket in the air; they make fine weather by shaking a small flat piece of wood attached to a stick by a string; and raise storms by strewing down on the ends of spruce branches. [14]

~ Because of their powers over the weather, twins are called the children of the sky and the woman who has given birth to twins is named 'Tilo' ('the sky'). ***South Africa***[14]

~ Spoil your twins and your whole family will prosper. ***Africa***

~ Parents of twins are so fertile they can increase the fertility of the plantain tree. Special ceremonies are held for this purpose. ***Central Africa***

~ When the twins are around eight days old, small basins containing food are set before them. The twins are then invoked to protect their parents from sickness, and to watch over them at all times. ***Africa***

~ Twins are so sociable that they didn't want to be born on their own.

~ The firstborn twin is more dominant and ambitious. The second twin is lazier, and will expect others to do his work all his life. ***UK***

~ There is always a good twin, and always an 'evil' twin. ***UK***
~ Wishes of twins are always fulfilled; therefore twins are feared and placated as they can harm those they hate. ***Tsimshian Indians: British Columbia***[14]
~ Many cultures assumed a man could father only one child at a time, so a mother giving birth to twins must have strayed or sinned somehow. Her children are therefore cursed. A typical story demonstrating this far-reaching belief is told about the man who mistrusted his wife. On an occasion, she gave birth to twins. His suspicions were not easily allayed, and he continued to rant about the twins, declaring he recognized one of them, but the other was a stranger. ***German Pennsylvania***
~ In some tribes, a man could have one of his testicles cut off so he'd not father twins again. ***South Africa***
~ Twins are transformed salmon. Therefore they must not go near water lest they turn back into fish. ***Kwatiutl Indians: British Columbia***[14]
~ If one twin dies, a wooden image is substituted for it in the cradle, alongside the living child so he doesn't miss the presence of his dead twin. The image is retained as a family fetish to ward off evil. ***The Benga Tribe: West Africa***
~ If both twins die, Mum must have two wooden images, and regard them as her living children; she worships them every morning by splitting kola nuts and throwing down a few drops of palm oil before them. ***Africa***
~ If one twin dies at birth, the other will inherit his dead sibling's strength.
~ When twins are born, if both of them are boys, the family have reformed for the better and there is rejoicing. A boy and a girl, however, forebode evil. ***India***
~ Twins, and the child born after twins called Dosu, are bad. ***Surinam***[37]
~ Twins are dreaded as an evil omen, and until recently were immediately put to death. As a punishment for having brought evil on her people, their mother was driven from the village to live alone in the forest. ***Calabar: West Africa***[38]
~ The second born of the twins is killed, but if the twins are of different sexes, the girl is killed. ***The Kobéwa Indians: Guyana***[21]
~ Twins were allowed to die or were deliberately killed by being enclosed in a pot or anthill. The birth of twins is an indication of the disfavour of the spirits, and possibly a punishment of adultery. Twin births are regarded as nonhuman, and their chi is the chi of an animal. After the birth of twins, a diviner is consulted to ascertain which spirit or ancestor had been offended, and sacrifice is offered to appease his wrath. ***Ibo Nigeria***[39]
~ Twins are a sign of dishonour. The mother is called names; some saying she is of the rodent family, as rats also have multiple births. When a woman gives birth to a baby and feels that another still remains, she'll bury the first rather than put up with her neighbour's jeers or her husband's reaction. The husband's view is that only one of the twins can possibly be his; the presence

Labour & Delivery

of the other is a sure sign of his wife's disloyalty. One of the Indian captains gives his wife a public whipping for daring to bring forth twins; and warns the other women of the serious beating he'll give them if they do the same. ***Saliva Indians Guyana*** [21]

~ The birth of triplets caused parents no uneasiness, but when quadruplets were born it was considered ill-omened. So when, in the principate of Augustus, a certain woman of low origin gave birth to two boys and two girls, it was believed to presage a famine which took place shortly afterward. ***Ancient Rome*** [16]

~ Although twins are welcomed, special ceremonies must be performed for the safety of the twin's lives, as they are at greater risk from evil. ***Gabun Africa*** [40]

OMENS RELATED TO THE NEWBORN'S LOOKS

~ Red-skinned babies will be fiery and hot-tempered.
~ The baby with a rash around the heart will be a healthy baby.
~ Little red Naevi marks on the skin are often referred to as 'stork marks' e.g.; where the stork caught hold of baby in its beak before delivering him.
~ A boy who looks like his mother will have good luck.
~ A pretty baby will be plain ugly when older. ***USA***
~ Babies with blue veins across their noses will not live to see twenty-one. ***Cornwall: UK***
~ A baby whose chin quivers will have a bad temper.
~ An 'innie' is considered a sign of a prosperous life for Baby, while an 'outie' is less lucky. ***China***

- **BIRTHMARKS**

~ If Baby has a birthmark on his head causing his hair to grow in blond, he's been kissed by a fairy (or an angel). Such kisses are very lucky.
~ A birthmark in the shape of a cross or dove indicates a blessed baby.
~ You can read birthmarks like tealeaves.
~ Birthmarks are the devil's mark, indicating where the devil was poking Baby in Mum's womb.
~ If the birthmark resembles a wheel, it's extremely lucky. The right side of the body is considered an even better omen than the left. ***India***
~ Birthmarks mark the sites of injuries gained in a previous life. ***New Age***
~ If Baby has a birthmark on his leg, he'll be hyperactive or travel far. A birthmark on the arm, is a sign of strength. A birthmark on the face, is a sign of beauty. ***Portugal***
~ A mole on Baby indicates future success.
~ 'If you've got a mole above your chin,
You'll never be beholden to any of your kin.' ***UK*** [5]

- **BABIES BORN WITH A CAUL**

~ The caul (or veil) is part of the foetal membrane that sometimes clings to the

head at birth when Mum's waters haven't broken.
~ The caul is a powerful aid in working magic. *UK*
~ The caul was retained as a talisman, usually placed in a locket around the child's neck. *(UK & Jewish)* or sewn into a tiny leather bag that must never be opened. *(Newfoundland)* If the caul is lost or discarded, Baby will become unlucky.
~ The fylgjar (guardian spirits) come into the world in the caul of a newborn child. If this caul is burnt or thrown away, Baby loses his guardian spirit for life. *Scandanavia* [9]
~ The caul should be carefully parched over a hot brick. Then a bit should be put into Baby's tea to prevent convulsions due to the irritation of a ghost. [31]
~ A baby born with a caul will be gifted with second sight *(Caribbean)* have the power to see Duppies without the Duppies harming him *(Jamaica*[31]*)* and will be strong in combating all evil spirits. Baby is thus given some of the dried powdered caul in water two or three days after birth. *(Haiti*[31]*)*
~ A Baby born in a caul will be intelligent, rich, travel much as an adult, and become a gifted speaker *(Belize)*. In Ancient Rome, lawyers purchased cauls to bring them luck while pleading.[41]
~ A child born with a caul will never drown. Cauls were therefore sold to Sailors for a lot of money. *UK*

- **EARS**

~ A baby will become a criminal if there is no crease between his earlobe and cheek.
~ A baby with wide and thick ears will live prosperously. *Chin*
~ Long ears are the dominant sign of wisdom and even immortality.
~ Big ears are a sign of future success. *Lincolnshire UK*

- **BABY'S FINAL EYE COLOUR**

~ If the child's eyebrows meet, it indicates a jealous or bad-tempered disposition. *UK*
~ 'Eyebrows that meet across the nose: Will never live to wear their wedding clothes'.[5]
~ Green eyes are devil's eyes, brown eyes are untrustworthy, blue eyes are kind. *UK*
~ Blue-eyed people possess the evil eye. *Mediterranean Countries*
~ Blue eyes say, 'Love me or I die', black eyes say, 'I Love me or I kill thee' and in Hindustani folklore, a blue-eyed girl is lucky. [5]
~ 'Grey-eyed greedy, Brown-eyed needy,
Black-eyed never likin', Till it shame a' its kin.' *UK* [5]
~ 'Blue-eyed beauty, Do your mother's duty;
Black eye, Brown eye,
Grey-eyed: greedy gut, Eat all the world up.' *Warwickshire UK* [5]

Labour & Delivery

~ *'Blue eye: beauty.*
Black eye; steal pie.
Grey eye; greedy gut.
Brown eye; love pie.' **Lincolnshire UK** [5]

- **FINGERS**

~ For a child to be born with an open hand is a sign of great generosity. If Baby clenches his fingers firmly, he'll be stingy. ***Turkey***

~ If Baby has big hands, he's predestined to be a manual worker. Long fingers indicate Baby has artistic and/or musical talents.

~ A child born with an extra toe or finger has lifelong luck.

- **HAIR**

~ Children born with long hair will die early unless the hair soon falls out. ***German Pennsylvania USA***

~ A baby born with a large amount of hair will have trouble in life. A lot of head hair indicates a lack of brains. In Victorian times, there was a popular proverb, 'Bush natural, more hairs than wit.' ***UK***

~ People with lots of body hair often have 'the evil eye'. ***Romany Gypsy***

~ A baby whose hair is long will live long. A hairy boy will be a future Romeo with the ladies.

~ If Baby is bald, he is sure to grow up quick-witted and intelligent. ***China***

~ A baby with more than one hair crown will be mischievous and disobedient. ***China***

~ Redheads will be fiery-tempered *(UK & USA)*, are unlucky, especially at New Year *(UK)*, and are to be feared *(Holland)*

~ Redheads are the devil's own and are untrustworthy; (Judas Iscariot was said to have had red hair[5]*)* and are held to be evil, malicious and unlucky, probably because Typhon, the evil principle, was red; therefore a red heifer was sacrificed to him by the Egyptians. [15]

~ Redheads are always born of an illicit affair, or as some say, are 'the milkman's' ***UK***

~ 'All the petty vices, all the lamentable shortcomings to which femininity is heir, have been laid to the charge of the reddish crown.' [5]

~ A red-haired girl is always self-conscious.

~ Red hair indicates good luck, and is called bálá kámeskro, or sun hairs. ***Romany Gypsy***[7]

~ Yellow hair was regarded in years gone by with ill favour and almost viewed a deformity.[5]

~ Children with curls might be fairies in disguise. Golden curls suggest mermaids, whereas elves are chocolate curled. Red curls are indicative of a witch, and raven curls indicate a very powerful fairy indeed. ***Scotland*** [5]

Baby Lore

- **LIPS**

~ Harelip is caused by Baby sucking his thumb in the womb.

~ Before a child is born, the angel Raphael teaches him all the seventy languages of the world; but as the child leaves his mother's womb, the same angel gives Baby a fillip on the upper lip causing him to forget them all again.
Russian Jews

~ A Cupid's bow lip means Baby will be a very loving, sensuous person.

- **TEETH**

~ A child born with teeth has syphilis (*UK*), will not live long (*German Pennsylvania*), or will become extremely selfish. For a girl to be born with teeth was considered ominous. (*Ancient Rome*[16])

~ A child born with teeth is regarded as a monster that will bring misfortune on his father, perhaps even devouring him. The child is therefore destroyed.
Ibo of Nigeria[42]

CHAPTER 14
TIMING IS EVERYTHING

THE DAY OF BIRTH

~ 'Monday's child is fair of face;
Tuesday's child is full of grace;
Wednesday's child is full of woe;
Thursday's child has far to go;
Friday's child is loving and giving;
Saturday's child works hard for a living.
But the child that is born on the Sabbath day
is fair and wise, good and gay.' ***UK***

~ 'Sunday's child is full of grace
Monday's child is full in the face
Tuesday's child is solemn and sad
Wednesday's child is merry and glad
Thursday's child is inclined to thieving
Friday's child is free in giving
Saturday's child works hard for a living' ***West Country Variant UK*** [12]

'Born on Monday, fair of face;
Born on Tuesday, full of grace;
Born on Wednesday, merry and glad;
Born on Thursday, wise and sad;
Born on Friday, Godly given;
Born on Saturday, earn a good living;
Born on Sunday, blithe and gay' ***Scotland***

'Sunday's child is full of grace,
Monday's child is fair of face;
Tuesday's child loves to race,
Wednesday's child is kind of heart;
Thursday's child is very smart,
Friday's child will never part;
Saturday's child is good of heart.' ***USA***

~ A baby born on one of the last days of the week will marry late or never. ***Estonia***[1]

Baby Lore

- **MONDAY'S CHILD**

~ The baby born on Monday will be gentle, serene, and truth loving. He'll have very strong convictions. *India*
~ Monday's child is wrathful. *Jewish* [2]
~ Monday's child is ruled by the Moon, Luna, and Artemis, and is impressionable, kind, adaptable, possessive, nurturing, and over-emotional.
~ Monday's colour is White

- **TUESDAY'S CHILD**

~ The baby born on Tuesday will simmer with anger. He'll excel, be brave, and be attractive to women. *India*
~ Tuesday's child is wealthy and sensual. *Jewish* [2]
~ Tuesday's child is ruled by Mars and Tiw and is courageous, strong, sporty, pioneering, independent, aggressive, hot-tempered, impatient, pushy, destructive and explosive.
~ Tuesday's colour is Red.

- **WEDNESDAY'S CHILD**

~ If born on Wednesday, Baby will be either stupid, or have a short life. *German Pennsylvania USA*
~ The baby born on Wednesday will be good-looking, intelligent, serious and studious. *India*
~ Wednesday's child will be intelligent and enlightened. *Jewish* [2]
~ Wednesday's child is ruled by Mercury, Hermes, and Wotan and is studious, intelligent, communicative, perceptive, versatile, healing, unreliable and careless.
~ Wednesday's colour is Purple.

- **THURSDAY'S CHILD**

~ The baby born on Thursday will be kind and compassionate. He'll be practical and a good timekeeper, hating to waste time. *India*
~ Thursday's child will be benevolent. *Jewish* [2]
~ Thursday's child is ruled by Jupiter, Zeus, and Thor, and is honourable, rich, fertile, generous, cheerful, philosophical, obsessive, conceited, hypocritical, sharp-tongued, and a traveller.
~ Thursday's colour is Blue.

- **FRIDAY'S CHILD**

~ Friday is a particularly bad day to begin anything on. It's very unlucky for a child to be born on a Friday, unless it's Good Friday. Whoever is born on a Friday must experience trouble. (*Austrian Tyrol* [3]) In Eastern Prussia, Sunday baptisms are thought to offset this bad luck. [3]
~ Babies born on Friday are practical and prefer to wear white clothes. *India*
~ Friday's child is pious. *Jewish* [2]
~ Children born on Friday are invulnerable to the assaults of the whole army

of hags and sorcerers. *Serbia* [3]
~ A baby born on Friday will be cheerful, passionate, light-hearted, and handsome. He'll delight in music, both vocal and instrumental, and will have a liking for fine clothes. Moreover, he'll be articulate in speech though of unstable character. *Italy* [3]
~ Friday's child is ruled by Venus and Freya and is affectionate, passionate, beautiful, seductive, oversexed, peaceful, caring, sociable, artistic, vain, vulgar and lazy.
~ Friday's Colour is Green.

- **SATURDAY'S CHILD**

~ Children born on Saturday tend to be slovenly, especially if birth occurs before the usual morning chores are finished about the house. *German Pennsylvania USA*
~ The baby born on a Saturday will become poor and skinny. He'll be overemotional and unwise in dealing with others. *India*
~ Saturday's child dies on the Sabbath. *Jewish* [2]
~ Saturday's child is ruled by Saturn and Kronus and is wise, professional, dedicated, practical, quiet, timid, miserable, suspicious, complaining and jealous.
~ Saturday's Colour is Black

- **SUNDAY'S CHILD**

~ Those born on Sunday will be talkative, brave and like to travel. *India*
~ Sunday's child is distinguished. *Jewish* [2]
~ Sunday's child is ruled by the Sun, Leo, and Apollo, and is creative, bold, noble, successful, outgoing, rich, healthy, loud, overbearing and egotistical.
~ Sunday's colour is Yellow.

HOUR OF BIRTH

~ Babies born in the morning can't see the spirit or fairy world. Those born at night, however, have power over ghosts and can see the spirits of the dead. *UK*
~ A child born early in the morning will always be lucky. *India*
~ A child born early in the morning had a better chance of survival. The saying was, 'the later the hour, the shorter the life'. *Scotland*
~ 'Chime children', born as the clock strikes the magical hours of three, six, nine and twelve are exceptionally lucky. They're insightful, able to see ghosts and talk to fairies without being harmed, have power over animals, and have knowledge of herb-lore. *UK*
~ Midnight-born babies have the gift of second sight. *UK*
~ It's unlucky for a child to be born at midday or at midnight. *India*
~ Children born between midnight on Friday and cockcrow on Saturday are seers, and have magical properties. *Somerset UK*
~ A child born at night will never see ghosts. *Scotland*

PLANETARY HOURS

~ If you want to find Baby's ruling planet, as per his birth hour, calculate this from the tables below. If Baby was born during the **daylight,** calculate his ruling planet by finding when sunrise was on that day. So for example, if sunrise at his place of birth was at 5.30am, then between 5.30am and 6.29am is the first planetary hour, 6.30am until 7.29am the second planetary hour and so on. Looking at the chart, we find that if he was born on Tuesday at 5.45am that makes him ruled by Mars. If he was born on Friday at 6.45am then he is ruled by Mercury. If Baby was born **after sunset**, use the second table to discover his planet, calculating in a similar way from the first hour of sunset. So if sunset was at 5.30pm, using the second chart we find Monday's child born at 5.45pm is ruled by Venus.

Day hours - from Sunrise to Sunset - the first hour of sunrise is ruled by the 'Hour 1' listed planet for that day and so on

Hour	Sun	Mon	Tues	Wed	Thurs	Fri	Sat
1	Sun	Moon	*Mars*	Mercury	Jupiter	Venus	Saturn
2	Venus	Saturn	Sun	Moon	Mars	*Mercury*	Jupiter
3	Mercury	Jupiter	Venus	Saturn	Sun	Moon	Mars
4	Moon	Mars	Mercury	Jupiter	Venus	Saturn	Sun
5	Saturn	Sun	Moon	Mars	Mercury	Jupiter	Venus
6	Jupiter	Venus	Saturn	Sun	Moon	Mars	Mercury
7	Mars	Mercury	Jupiter	Venus	Saturn	Sun	Moon
8	Sun	Moon	Mars	Mercury	Jupiter	Venus	Saturn
9	Venus	Saturn	Sun	Moon	Mars	Mercury	Jupiter
10	Mercury	Jupiter	Venus	Saturn	Sun	Moon	Mars
11	Moon	Mars	Mercury	Jupiter	Venus	Saturn	Sun
12	Saturn	Sun	Moon	Mars	Mercury	Jupiter	Venus

Night Hours - from Sunset to Sunrise

Hour	Sun	Mon	Tues	Wed	Thurs	Fri	Sat
1	Jupiter	*Venus*	Saturn	Sun	Moon	Mars	Mercury
2	Mars	Mercury	Jupiter	Venus	Saturn	Sun	Moon
3	Sun	Moon	Mars	Mercury	Jupiter	Venus	Saturn
4	Venus	Saturn	Sun	Moon	Mars	Mercury	Jupiter
5	Mercury	Jupiter	Venus	Saturn	Sun	Moon	Mars
6	Moon	Mars	Mercury	Jupiter	Venus	Saturn	Sun
7	Saturn	Sun	Moon	Mars	Mercury	Jupiter	Venus
8	Jupiter	Venus	Saturn	Sun	Moon	Mars	Mercury
9	Mars	Mercury	Jupiter	Venus	Saturn	Sun	Moon
10	Sun	Moon	Mars	Mercury	Jupiter	Venus	Saturn
11	Venus	Saturn	Sun	Moon	Mars	Mercury	Jupiter
12	Mercury	Jupiter	Venus	Saturn	Sun	Moon	Mars

DATE OF BIRTH

~ Unlucky Days in each month. Whoever is born on these days is unfortunate and suffers much poverty.

January 1, 2, 3, 4, 6, 11, 12.
February 1, 17, 18.
March 14, 16.
April 10, 17, 18.
May 7, 8.
June 17.
July 17, 21.
August 20, 21.
September 10, 18.
October 6.
November 6, 10.
December 6, 11, 15. ***Germany*** [24]

~ The unlucky Days according to the opinion of certain Astronomers: [43]
January 1, 2, 4, 5, 10, 15, 17, 29, **very unlucky**
February 26, 27, 28, **unlucky**; 8, 10, 17, **very unlucky**
March 16, 17, 20 **very unlucky**
April 7, 8, 10, 20 **unlucky**; 16, 21, very unlucky
May 3, 6, **unlucky**; 7, 15, 20, **very unlucky.**
June 10, 22, **unlucky**; 4, 8, **very unlucky**
July 15, 21, **very unlucky**
August 1, 29, 30, **unlucky**; 19, 20, **very unlucky**
September 3, 4, 21, 23, **unlucky**; 6, 7, **very unlucky**
October 4, 16, 24, **unlucky**; 6 **very unlucky**
November 5, 6, 29, 30, **unlucky**; 15, 20, **very unlucky**
December, 15, 22, **unlucky**; 6, 7, 9, **very unlucky**

~ A child born on the thirteenth will be unlucky. ***German Pennsylvania USA***
~ All children born on the thirteenth of any month are under the protection of Santa Lucia. ***Italy***
~ Those conceived or born on February 29th are especially lucky. ***UK***
~ Good Friday babies will have sadness all their lives. ***UK***
~ A child born on Good Friday and baptised on Easter Sunday has a gift of healing. If a boy, he should go into the ministry. ***UK***
~ Easter babies will be joyous and energetic and are ensured a lucky life. ***UK***
~ Children born on April Fools' Day are lucky in everything but gambling. ***UK***
~ A child born at Whitsuntide will have an evil temper, and may commit a murder. To turn away ill-luck from a child born at that time, a grave must be dug and the infant laid in it for a few minutes. After this process the evil spell is broken, and the child is safe. ***Ireland*** [15]
~ A baby born on Halloween can see and speak to spirits.
~ Children born on Halloween will enjoy lifelong protection against evil spirits and will have second sight. ***USA***
~ A girl born on Christmas Eve will become a witch and a boy will become a werewolf. ***Italy***
~ The child born on Christmas Day will have a special fortune (*Scotland*) and

is protected against drowning or hanging. He will be blessed with many talents, and will become generous. Brighter than others are, he can hear and understand 'cattle talk' and can see ghosts. (*German Pennsylvania*)

~ Those born on Christmas Day will never encounter a ghost, nor will they have anything to fear from spirits.

~ It's lucky to be born on New Year's Day. **UK**

~ The child born on New Year's Day will have the gifts of foresight *and* hindsight.

MONTH OF BIRTH

~ A person born in January can see ghosts. **German Pennsylvania**

~ April babies make unpredictable people.

~ Babies born in May are usually sickly and never do really well. 'All the May bairns die and decay,' (*Scotland*[5]) Children born in May are called 'May Chets.' Kittens born in May are destroyed as 'May Chets, Bad luck begets'. Another saying is 'A hot May, fat Church hay,' meaning many funerals as a consequence. (*Cornwall: UK* [12])

~ June babies will never be sleepy heads. **African-American**

~ September babies will never have any luck unless they wear garnets.

~ The month of Safar is a month of ill fortune. Because of the various evil omens attached to this month, some Muslims regard the first thirteen days of this month to be specifically evil and bad luck to be born in. **Islamic**

OTHER

~ It was very unlucky for a child to be born at low-water spring tide. He'd never prosper and if he was an heir to land or property, he'd be sure to destroy it. *Isle of Man* [44]

~ At whatever state of the tide Baby was born, whether low or high, flowing or ebbing, that's the way it will be when the child eventually dies. *Isle of Man* [44]

~ Spring babes will bloom and grow, being full of joy whereas winter babes will be more depressed and lazier as adults. **UK**

~ 'Red dawning, cloudy sky, Bloody death shalt thou die.' **Romany Gypsy** [7]

THE MOON'S INFLUENCE

~ A child born at the interval between the old and new moons is fated to die before reaching puberty. **Cornwall: UK**

~ Babies born at or near the new moon will never do any good in the world. **UK**

~ Children born in the full of the moon, are stronger and larger than those born in the wane. **UK** [45]

~ 'Full moon, high sea; great man thou shalt be.' A child born at full moon will also make a happy marriage. **Romany Gypsy** [7]

BABY'S STARS

~ A boy who is born in Pisces is usually thirsty. *German Pennsylvania*
~ A boy born in the Venus-morningstar gets a wife much younger than himself; if born in the Venus-eveningstar he'll get one much older. The opposite applies to baby girls. *Germany* [1]
~ If born under the influence of Venus, Baby will become rich and adulterous.
~ A boy is extremely lucky to be born under the star, Moola. However, a Moola girl will be very unlucky. *India*
~ A baby born under Kartik is unlucky, but if he is born early in the morning, this cancels it out and he'll always be lucky. *India*
~ Boys born under Chitrai make their fathers beggars, boys born under Rohini bring bad luck to their uncles, and a grandfather may rather die than hear his grandson's star is Kettai. *India*
~ A boy born under Swati and a girl born under Pooradam is very unlucky. *India*
~ A girl born under the Avittam star will find gold even in a pot of bran. *India*
~ A child born under Uttradam brings luck to the field and crops, and the baby born under Bharani will rule the earth. *India*

OTHER ASTROLOGY

~ As so much has been written in other places on Astrology, there is little need to go into much detail here. As well as the Gregorian astrology system (Taurus, Libra etc) there is also the Chinese, Indian Vedic, & Celtic systems. I have included very basic information on the Vedic & Celtic systems here so those wishing to may do further research into their baby's signs elsewhere.

- **INDIAN VEDIC RASHIS (SIGNS)**

December 21 - January 21: Makara
January 21 - February 21: Kumbha
February 21 - March 21: Mina
March 21 - April 21: Mesha
April 21 - May 21: Vrishabha
May 21 - June 21: Mithuna
June 21 - July 21: Karkata
July 21 - August 21: Simha
August 21 - September 21: Kanya
September 21 - October 21: Tula
October 21 - November 21: Vrischika
November 21 - December 21: Dhanur

- **CELTIC ASTROLOGY**

December 24 – January 20: Beth (The Birch Tree)
Ruled by the Sun and Lugh, the Warrior god and inventor of arts and crafts
January 21 – February 17: Luis (The Rowan Tree)

Ruled by Uranus and Brigid, the goddess of fertility and poetry
February 18 – March 17: Nuin (The Ash Tree)
Ruled by Neptune and the Magician, storyteller and trickster
March 18 – April 14: Fearn (The Alder Tree)
Ruled by Mars and Bran the Blessed, the god of the spirit world
April 15 – May 12; Saille (The Willow Tree)
Ruled by the Moon and Ceridwen, the Moon goddess
May 13 – June 9; Huatha (The Hawthorn Tree)
Ruled by Vulcan and Olwen, the summer flower maiden
June 10 – July 7; Duir (The Oak Tree)
Ruled by Jupiter and The Dagda, Father of all Gods
July 8 – August 4; Tinne (The Holly Tree)
Ruled by Earth and Govannon, the Smith God
August 5 – September 1; Colle (The Hazel Tree)
Ruled by Mercury and Manannan Mac Lir, the Sea god, a master of disguise
September 2 – September 29 Muin (The Vine Tree/Blackberry)
Ruled by Venus and the Tuatha De Danaan Gods of Light
September 30 – October 27; Gort (The Ivy Tree)
Ruled by the Moon or Persephone and Guinevere, the fairy bride
October 28 – November 24; Ngetal (The Reed Tree)
Ruled by Pluto and Pwyll, the God of the Underworld
November 25 – December 23; Ruis (The Elder Tree)
Ruled by Saturn and Cailleach Beara, the crown goddess and Celtic tribal mother

Numerology

The Life Path Number is calculated from the birth date and represents the inherent traits Baby will carry with him through life.

Convert the day of birth to a single digit, convert the month to a single digit, then convert the total digits of the year and reduce this sum to a single digit. The individual digits representing the month, day, and year, are then added together to reduce the sum once again to a single digit.

E.g.: If Baby was born on September 28, 2004, add the day 28 (2+8 = 10, which is reduced to 1) to the month (9) to the year 2004 (which reduces to 6). Thus the total of the month, day, and year is 1+9+6 = 16   1 + 6 = 7

This date means a number 7 Life path individual. Once this number has been assessed, Baby's name can be numerologically selected to help make up for any deficiencies in his Life Path. (For more on numerology, see page 169)

PART IV
THE NEWBORN
& NEW PARENTS

Chapter 15
The Newborn

~ Newborns that made no sound were rubbed with the afterbirth. *Jewish*
~ If Baby has difficulties breathing, scorch his forehead with a hot needle. *India*
~ Baby is given catnip to 'hive' out the bad entity all babies are born with that can kill them if left untreated. *African American*
~ A little roast pig was given to a newborn to cure him of all his Mother's Longings during pregnancy. *17th Century England*
~ Newborns are steamed or rubbed with oils to make them stronger. Sometimes the mothers are steamed too. *Aborigine*
~ After Baby is born, a few drops of mustard oil are put on his nostrils, ears and tongue. *Bangladesh*
~ Boiled water and honey is given to Baby for his first two days, then he's put onto Mum's breast. *Ancient Rome*
~ To make a baby's birthmark disappear, immediately smear it with his afterbirth.
~ Wash the Newborn's face in an egg to make his skin soft. *USA*
~ Premature babies were fully wrapped in cotton wool and placed in an incubator with three hot water bottles. This is probably where the expression 'can't keep them wrapped up in cotton wool' originates. *Edwardian UK* [27]
~ A newborn isn't placed immediately into his mother's arms, but first laid at her feet, so her left foot may touch his mouth so he'll not be rebellious. *Estonia*[1]
~ Immediately after birth, Baby is bathed, rubbed with salt for protection, and wrapped in swaddling clothes. *Jewish*
~ A new baby is immediately swaddled tightly and should only be handled by his mother to maintain a state of 'wuzho'. *Romany Gypsy*
~ The gentle handling of a newborn gives it feelings of great discomfort; therefore all unnecessary movements should be avoided. *Edwardian UK* [27]
~ Don't lay a newborn on his left side first, or he'll always be awkward.
~ Blowing into a newborn's mouth causes him to be pleasant in later life. *Turkey*
~ When a boy is born, let his feet push against his father's breast, and he'll not come to a bad end. *Germany* [1]
~ As soon as a girl is born, seat her on her mother's breast, and say, 'God make thee a good woman' and she'll never slip or come to shame. *France* [1]
~ A pinch of pollen is put on Baby's tongue for strong lungs and steady growth. (*Navajo Tribe USA*) and consecrated Haoma juice so he might have

The Newborn & New Parents

wisdom and knowledge. (*Zoroastrian*) [23]

~ Newborns were passed through a wolf skin in order to be 'born of the She-Wolf.' ***Slavic***

~ Rub a little honey on Baby's head for luck (*Wales*) or spit on him to secure health and long life. (*Ireland*)

~ At the birth of a child, everyone present takes a stone and throws it behind him, saying, 'This into the jaws of the Streghoi' (evil spirits and witches) ***Romanian Romany Gypsy*** [7]

~ The first time Baby is taken out of the labour room, he must be taken upstairs or he'll not go to heaven. ***Pennsylvania USA***

~ Baby should be carried upstairs rather then down on leaving the labour room to ensure he 'rises' in life. Where there are no stairs, midwives should climb onto furniture placed in the doorway to satisfy this requirement. If this isn't done, Baby is doomed to a lowly life. ***UK & USA***

~ A child on his first day should be carried to the attic and allowed to look out the window if he's to become a respected citizen. ***German Pennsylvania***

~ Put a silver spoon or Bible within Baby's hand, and then carry him to the attic. This must be done before he's nine days old. ***USA***

~ A child will receive lofty thoughts if a louse is placed upon his head and he's carried to the upper story of the house, before he is nine days old. ***Fayette County USA***

~ When witches are attached to any family or place, they secretly enter the house and carry the cradle with Baby up to the attic. Then the witch takes the sack of the cradle, lays the babe on it, and puts at his head coarse salt, and an open Bible at his feet. Then four gold chains and four gold rings are put, one in every corner of the bed, and two lighted candles are placed at Baby's head. Then with the chains, the bed is hung to the rafters with Baby in it, and the witch repeats:

'*This for myself I have not done,*
But for love to this little one,
Not because his family
Great or wealthy chance to be.
But that he may rise, have I
Brought him to this room so high;
Thus may he by talents thrive,
And be the greatest man alive!' ***Italy*** [46]

~ What a baby first clutches at shows his favourite occupation. (*Estonia*[1]) Let Baby touch a baseball so he'll become a great ball player. (*Puerto Rico*) A pencil put into Baby's hands makes him good-natured and studious. (*Turkey*)

~ Baby is held to the sky, and someone says, 'Behold the only thing greater than yourself' to empower him. It tells Baby of all he can be, and the wonders of the universe. ***Pagan***

~ A man jumps over the baby. If he lands safely, Baby will pass safely through childhood. ***Burgos Spain***

~ A baby's first cradle is a tray on which a bit of iron and a peck of unhusked rice is laid. When the baby is promoted from this tray, the rice on which he has lain is measured to tell his future; if the measure is brimming, he'll be rich; if it's short, poor; the balance of the rice is thrown to the chicken to avert bad luck ***Perak Malaysia*** [22]

~ Let Baby suck at a towel dipped in cockroach's excretion, to help get rid of meconium stool. ***Thailand***

~ A bottle of whisky is bought to, 'Wet the child's head' and bring good luck. It was not uncommon for Baby's first drink to be whisky, immediately fed to him on a teaspoon. Whiskey was regarded as 'an infallible cure for all infantile ailments.' To ensure good luck, this teaspoon should be silver. However, most households could not afford this luxury, so a silver coin, often borrowed, was placed in a normal spoon instead. ***Orkney Islands*** [6]

~ Every new life is seen as a carrier of light, so for the first forty days a bright light burns day and night in Baby's home. ***Malaysia***

~ During the first six weeks, don't take Baby inside your cloak, or he'll be gloomy, and always meet with sorrow. ***Germany*** [1]

~ Every newborn is greeted with a handshake by everyone, even the children, to ensure he is a well-liked member of the community. ***Inuit Eskimo***

~ Flowers are put into water and the Newborn bathed in it. The flowers are subsequently taken out, dried and kept among the child's clothes until the next baby arrives. ***Malaysia*** [20]

~ A medicine-man conjures a newborn's soul into a coconut-half, which he covers with a cloth and places on a square platter or charger suspended by cords from the roof. This is to place the child's soul in a safer place than his own frail little body. ***The Dyaks of Pinoeh: South-east Borneo*** [14]

~ An empty coconut, split and spliced together again, hangs beside a rough wooden image of an ancestor. The baby's soul is believed to be temporarily deposited in the coconut so he may be safe from evil spirits; but when the child grows bigger and stronger, the soul will take up its permanent abode in his own body. ***Kei Islands*** [14]

BABY GIFTS

~ Traditional presents to newborns included matches, fire being an ancient charm against the supernatural. These were pinned into the child's long clothes. Matches also 'lit the child on his way to heaven.' ***East Riding of Yorkshire*** [9]

~ Eggs, symbolising fertility are boiled hard, then dyed red, to bring Baby good luck (*China*) A gift of eggs symbolises the child's fertility and

immortality. (*UK*[9])
~ It's customary to give an egg (representative of the trinity with its three parts; the shell, the yolk and the white), salt and some bread. **Northern England**
~ If Baby is given a newly-laid egg, piece of bread and a pinch of salt he'll always have the essentials of life. **Scotland**
~ Salt, a symbol of immortality and eternal life, and protection from evil, was amongst the first gifts given to a baby. (*Pagan*) The gift of salt signifies salubrity of mind and body. (*UK*[9])
~ A gift of white bread represents all the necessities of life. *UK*[9]
~ On her way home from Church, let Mum buy bread and lay it in the cradle so her child will have bread as long as he lives. **Germany**[1]
~ A gift of a silver spoon put into a newborn's mouth makes him rich, hence the expression 'born with a silver spoon in the mouth'. **UK**
~ Godparents should buy the child a spoon, lest he learn to dribble. **Germany**[1]
~ Socks, slippers, or shoes are unlucky gifts. **Philippines**
~ Gifts are given and accepted only with the right hand. **India**
~ To ensure good fortune, be sure Baby's first gift is a silver coin. Place it into the child's hand; if the child drops the coin, he'll have difficulty holding onto money throughout life, and if he grasps it tightly; he'll be fortunate with money. There's the tale of a notoriously mean Scotsman who went to see his first great grandchild taking a gift of a gold sovereign with him. The baby grasped the coin tightly and the old man was delighted as this meant the baby would have a good grasp of what mattered. If the child had let go the coin, it was said he'd have grown up generous.
~ Visitors would rarely leave without handing over a silver coin saying, 'I'll have to give the bairn a luck penny'. **Scotland**
~ Crossing a baby's palm with silver fends off evil spirits.
~ The godparent's 'chrism-gift' consisted of a two or three meter linen cloth and a gift of money. The chrism was placed under Baby's pillow to help him become rich.
~ The Godfather's money makes Baby rich and lucky.
~ Give Baby a red coral and silver bell teething ring. The coral wards off the evil eye, and the silver bells bring good fortune and drive off evil.
~ If a man visits a woman during confinement and his hat is thrown on the bed, it will not be returned to him until he has given a present for the newborn. **German Pennsylvania**
~ Used merchandise can be dangerous. You don't know where it's been or how holy the previous owners were, so it could have a demon attached to it. **Jehovah's Witness**
~ To give a child an opal, unless he's born in October, will bring bad luck.
~ If a stranger wants to see Baby, he must give a gift to the baby. **Bulgaria**

~ If the child is a boy, a spade is buried and unearthed when the child is eleven years old so he'll be blessed with work. *The Andes*
~ In rich families, a pen and pencil were given to Baby hoping he'd become a good student and subsequently a clerk or author. *Russia*

CEREMONIES FOR THE NEW BABY

~ The father prays for intelligence, strength, and beauty for his child and applies a minuscule portion of ground rice and barley mixed with ghee on the newborn's tongue. The rice and barley are to be hand-ground by either a pregnant woman or a virgin girl. *Hindi*

~ The 'Jatakarma' sacrament is performed before the umbilical cord is cut. After showering, the father touches his baby's lips with a gold spoon or ring dipped in honey, curds, and ghee. The word 'vak' (speech) is whispered three times into Baby's right ear, and the Ayusya rite is performed to give Baby a long life. *Hindi*

~ The custom of pronouncing the creed in the Newborn's right ear and the call to prayer in the left is to protect Baby from his evil Qarin twin. *Islamic*

~ The day after birth, the 'Medhajanana' ceremony is held to give intelligence to the baby. The father gives his baby a little honey and ghee. He does this with his ring finger, ensuring he is wearing a gold ring on it. Ghee helps mental development, memory, talent, and removes hysteria, headache, and epilepsy. With each feeding Dad utters one word of the Gayatri mantra, namely; 'Bhu' with the first feeding: 'Bhuvah' with the second feeding; 'Svah' with the third feeding; 'Bhur Bhuvah Svah' with the fourth feeding. *Hindi*

~ Seven days (in some places, fourteen days or twenty one days) after birth, at the Aqiqah (naming) ceremony, two goats or ewes for a boy and one goat or ewe for a girl are sacrificed to ransom Baby from hell. *Islamic*

~ On the seventh day, the child's hair is shaved in a ceremony called Moondun, and gold or silver equal to the weight of the shaved hair (or the equivalent to the price of the metals) is donated to the poor. The shaved hair is tied up in a piece of cloth buried under the earth or thrown into the river. Some launch it out on a raft illuminated by lamps, after putting flour, sugar, ghee, and milk, over the hair. *Islamic*

~ Twenty days after birth, the soft spot on Baby's head is beginning to close. The parents scatter cornmeal on Baby's head and then in all four directions to attract the kachina, who following the trail of cornmeal come to Baby and give him the wisdom of the gods. Once the head has closed, the child is on his own. *Hopi Tribe USA*

~ A white corn representing Mother Earth is placed next to the Newborn. After twenty days, the ear of the corn is rubbed over Baby to bless him in the naming ceremony. This ritual is repeated when he's twenty-one, and is given a

new name to be used for the rest of his life. ***Hopi Tribe USA***
~ A 'Redemption of the Firstborn' is held on Baby's thirtieth day. Traditionally, this was done only for a firstborn male not born by caesarean section. This ceremony ritualistically redeems or 'buys' Baby from a lifetime of priestly service by paying money to a priest who then passes the money onto charity. ***Jewish***
~ Baby's parents have a large party to celebrate the first month birthday. Offerings are presented to the 'Holy Godmother', thanking her for protecting the child. During the ceremony, a flower wet with special water from the altar is dripped into Baby's mouth to ensure he learns to speak sweetly scented words. ***Vietnam***
~ After forty-four days, Baby is introduced to 'Mother Earth'. The midwife carries the baby to the top of the stairs, recites incantations and marks a cross on the soles of Baby's feet with lime. She descends and then puts the child's feet on iron, a tray containing gold and silver, and then the earth. Baby is then carried down to the river to meet 'Father Water'. A candle is lit and the mother and midwife wash each others hair. An offering is made to the water spirit and Baby is passed through incense smoke. Then a live fowl is placed in the water and Baby made to tread on it, so he has power over all domestic animals. Next a sprouting coconut seedling is set afloat and his feet are placed on it, so he has power over all food plants. Lastly a jungle sapling is put in the stream and setting his feet upon it gives Baby dominion over the forest. ***Perak: Malaysia***[22]
~ Karnavedha (ear piercing) ceremony. The child's ears are pierced for protection from hernia and other diseases and also for decoration. ***Hindi***

PLANTING A TREE

~ At the birth of a child, a tree is planted. The tree, it's hoped, will grow with the child, and is tended with special care. ***Europe & Russia***[14]
~ An apple tree is planted for a boy and a pear tree for a girl, the belief being that the child will flourish or dwindle with the tree. ***Aargau Switzerland***[14]
~ A newborn's life is united with a tree's life by driving a pebble into the bark. This is supposed to give them complete mastery over the child's life; if the tree is cut down, the child will die. ***Papua New Guinea***[14]
~ When two children are born on the same day, people plant two trees of the same kind and dance round them. The life of each child is believed to be bound up with the life of one of the trees; and if the tree dies or is thrown down, the child will soon die. ***Benga Tribe West Africa***[14]
~ A fruit tree is planted for a baby, and the child's fate is bound up with that of the tree's. If the tree shoots up rapidly, it will go well with the child; but if the tree is dwarfed or shrivelled, nothing but misfortune can be expected for Baby. ***Borneo***[14]

~ The Romans, in common with many other peoples, ancient and modern, often identified the lifetime of a particular tree with the duration of the life of the person at whose birth it was planted. So on the country estate of the Flavians stood an ancient oak which sent forth a branch on each of the three occasions when Vespasia gave birth. *Ancient Rome*

~ Near the Castle of Dalhousie, not far from Edinburgh, there grows an oak tree, called the Edgewell Tree, which is popularly believed to be linked to the fate of the family by a mysterious tie; for they say when one of the family dies, or is about to die, a branch falls from the Edgewell Tree. Thus, on seeing a great bough drop from the tree on a quiet, still day in July 1874, an old forester exclaimed, 'The laird's deid noo!' and soon after news came that Fox Maule, eleventh Earl of Dalhousie, was dead. *Scotland* [14]

DRESSING THE NEWBORN

~ Wrap a little bread and salt in Baby's swaddling for protection. *Germany* [1]

~ Put an old (cloth) nappy (diaper) on the newborn, so he doesn't become a thief. *USA*

~ Put an old nappy on a newborn, or he can't stool easily. *German Pennsylvania*

~ Burn the first nappy for luck. *German Pennsylvania*

~ A baby's first nappy should not be left out to dry when the moon is up for fear of attracting its malignant influence.

~ A woman will not have chloasma if she wipes her face with the first nappy wetted by her newborn child. *German Pennsylvania*

~ Don't wring dry a cloth nappy, or Baby's body will become twisted. *Thailand*

~ The baby's first stool is smeared on Mum's face. *Navajo Tribe USA*

~ Mum must not show signs of disgust if Baby soils himself during a nappy change. *Navajo Tribe*

~ A dirty face and black clothes are a baby's protection against evil spirits. *India*

~ The first time a baby is dressed, the clothes must be put on over his feet, not his head. *UK*

~ Deduct nothing from the cost of making a child's first dress; the more you scrimp, the less luck he'll have. *Germany* [1]

~ The first dress put on a child should be new; an old one will cause him to be a 'slop'. *German Pennsylvania*

~ If a new outfit's worn for the first time on a Sunday, or when going to church, it will wear twice as long. *German Pennsylvania*

~ If Baby is dressed up fine on his first three Sundays, his clothes will sit well on him in the future. *Germany* [1]

~ The Newborn is dressed in old clothes for fear evil spirits will be jealous of the new clothes and cause Baby to become ill. After the one month ceremony, it's okay to dress Baby in new clothes. ***Vietnam***

~ The first time Baby is carried out, let a garment be put on him inside-out. ***Germany*** [1]

~ Dress the child in the opposite sex's clothes and you will thwart the devil by confusing him. Some mothers continued to dress their boys in petticoats and their girls in trousers up until the age of fourteen. ***Ireland***

~ Dressing boys in girls' clothes until they were ten years of age was a means of tricking the fairies, who were always on the lookout for healthy young boys. ***UK & Ireland***

~ The Roman child up to the age of puberty needed the protection of a special purple bordered dress which possessed religious significance. ***Ancient Rome*** [16]

~ Low dresses and short sleeves expose the lungs to chill as the lungs extend above the collarbone and come down under the armpits. ***Edwardian UK*** [27]

~ It's good luck to put clothes on inside-out. If you accidentally put clothes on inside-out, you must not correct it that day, lest you take the good luck away. ***Europe***

~ If you put something on inside out, cast it to the floor and step on it before putting it back on the right way. ***Russia***

~ Keep a baby in socks to avoid all sorts of medical problems.

~ Babies were bound head to foot with yards of material like a mummy, their arms fixed to their sides. They were then placed on a pillow and carried around like a parcel. ***19th Century Italy***

~ Always place Baby's right arm in the right sleeve first. If you want to prevent headache or toothache, you must also form the habit of putting on the right stocking, first, and the right shoe first. ***German Pennsylvania***

COLOURS OF CLOTHES

~ Fairies and other malicious wood spirits are said to wear green, and anyone who wears green or otherwise favours the colour will come under the fairies' evil influence.

~ It's unlucky for a baby to wear green as the fairies might steal him away. ***Ireland***

~ Anyone who wears green will have to wear black soon afterwards (i.e.: someone will soon die). ***UK***

~ Boys dressed in pink will become effeminate, girls in blue, butch.

~ Red and green should never be seen. ***Scotland***

~ Orange can over-stimulate Baby. Brown can 'earth' an excitable baby.

~ Baby will be depressed wearing dark colours.

~ Black colours represent males and blue colours, females. ***Navajo Tribe USA***

~ Blue is the most sacred colour and is used to honour gods. ***Hopi Tribe USA***

~ Here are some of the other meanings attached to colours:

Black; night, underworld, male, cold, disease, death
Blue; sky, water, female, clouds, lightning, moon, thunder, sadness
Red; wounds, sunset, thunder, blood, earth, war, day
Yellow; sunshine, day, dawn
White; winter, death, snow
Green; plant life, earth, summer, rain. **Native American**

WASHING CLOTHES BELIEFS

~ To find a louse on linen is a sign of sickness. To find two lice, means the sickness is severe. Three is an omen to prepare for a death. **Cornwall UK** [12]
~ Baby's underwear can't be hanged out following afternoon Prayer. **Turkey**
~ Baby clothes left outside until sunset causes Baby to be bewitched. **Turkey**
~ Never leave Baby's clothes outside at night lest they the clothes become bewitched. **Kyrgyzstan**
~ If clothes are left hanging out until sunset, he that puts them on will bewitch everybody. **Germany** [1]
~ 'They that wash Monday got all the week to dry
They that wash Tuesday are pretty nearby
They that wash Wednesday make a good housewife
They that wash Thursday must wash for their life
They that wash Friday mush wash indeed
They that wash Saturday are sluts indeed.' **Cornwall UK** [12]
~ If Mum washes on New Year's Day, she'll wash her family away. **UK**
~ It is unlucky to wash anything on Saturday.
~ Wash your linen, by the waning moon so the dirt may disappear with the dwindling light.[1]

BELIEFS RE: BABY'S SEX

~ A boy is welcomed into the world with the words: 'A boy is born to the world; a blessing has come into the world' but at a girl's birth, the walls are said to weep. When a boy is born, he brings peace to the world, whereas a girl brings nothing. **Jewish**
~ Baby boys are found in the cabbage patch, baby girls amongst the roses. **France**
~ A daughter born after other girls is called 'Kamaria' meaning 'enough'. **Jewish** [2]
~ A couple with only girls must have sinned and are being punished. **Vietnam**
~ If a woman has only boys, it's a sign of war; if only girls, a sign of peace. **Estonia**[1]
~ Girl babies come from the Isle of May and boy babies come from the Bass Rock. **East Coast of Scotland**

The Newborn & New Parents

CHAPTER 16
ADVICE FOR NEW PARENTS

~ Mum must keep warm at all costs staying out of cold drafts. (*China*) Mum should sleep on a special bed next to the fireplace for this reason. (*India*)
~ Mum should wrap up well and then lie in the open air or before a large open window for a few hours each day. ***Edwardian UK*** [27]
~ The things touched by a new Mum kill those who handle them. New mums are forbidden under pain of death to touch anything men use, or even to walk on a path any man frequents. All vessels used by them during their confinement period are burned. ***Aborigine Australia*** [14]
~ The pots which a woman touches, while the impurity of childbirth is on her, should be destroyed; spears and shields defiled by her touch must be purified. ***Uganda*** [14]
~ The new mum shouldn't read or watch television as it harms her vision. ***Philippines***
~ Mum should close or cross her legs during the first few weeks to reduce the amount of air entering her body. Too much air results in bleeding and/or a permanently fat abdomen. ***Ghana***
~ Neither fire, salt or bread may be given away from the house of a woman during the first six weeks following childbirth. ***Germany*** [1]

CONFINEMENT OF MOTHER & CHILD

~ The term 'confinement' was to be taken literally. By general consensus, most nations agreed on a period of forty days. Mother or Baby shouldn't leave the house during their confinement period, except perhaps to go to the baptism service which was normally performed when the baby was between one and two weeks old.
~ Don't take Baby outside for the first seven days lest bad luck is brought on him. ***Umbundu People Angola***
~ Baby shouldn't leave the house until he's one month old, so jealous people can't give him the 'evil eye'. ***Portugal***
~ Baby mustn't be shown to a stranger until he's at least forty days old. ***Slavic***
~ No family member may enter Mum or Baby's room for the first forty nights. ***Romany Gypsy***
~ Never take unbaptised children on journeys or they may be abducted by fairies.
~ Mum is expected to stay at the place where she gave birth for seven days to protect Baby from evil spirits. Mum is also very vulnerable during this time since unclean spirits are fond of polluted blood and breast milk. If Mum leaves her labour room to go to toilet, she covers her hair, takes a piece of metal, and

sprinkles her path with water in order to banish dangers in front of her. Before re-entering the room, Mum walks around a fire pot and warms her hands and feet to expel any bad spell which might have attached to her outside. Mum is allowed to leave the labour room on the seventh day. However, she remains polluted as long as her bleeding continues. ***Muslim Bangladesh***
~ The dai (midwife) and barber remove childbirth pollution. The number of days of pollution varies in different caste groups. Brahmans perform purifying rituals once on the 11th day, while Sudras perform them on the 3rd, 11th, and 30th days. During the ritual, Mum and Baby take baths, and Baby's hair and nails are cut. They then wear new clothes discarding whatever they used during their seclusion period due to birth pollution. Mum is then fed ghee, honey, milk, gangajal (sacred water from the Ganges) and go-chona (a bit of cow dung and a few drops of cow's urine). Then she's given a meal consisting of five dishes. She's then allowed to leave the labour room, but is still considered polluted for a certain period. ***Hindi Bangladesh***
~ Mum is laid on a platform and toasted frequently during forty-four days of seclusion. The men dread the contagion of the woman's effeminacy, weakness, timidity and hysteria at this time. When the forty-four days of purification are complete, the midwife throws away the platform on which Mum has been roasted, and the ashes of the fire that has burnt without cease by her side. ***Malaysia*** [22]
~ Mum is secluded for two to three weeks in a temporary hut erected on sacred ground; during this time she's forbidden from touching food, and is even fed by someone else. If anyone touches Baby during this period, that person is also made 'taboo' until Mum's purification ceremony is performed. ***Tahiti*** [14]
~ Mum and Baby are separated from the main camp, and live alone in a 'moon house' for a full lunar cycle after birth. ***Native American***
~ Mum is isolated from the camp for one month if she has a boy and for two months if she has a girl. ***Inuit Eskimo***
~ Mum is unclean for three weeks after birth, so she must stay in her room with Baby. A hole is dug in the corner as her toilet. After thirty days of seclusion, relatives and friends gather for a celebration where gifts are given to the baby. ***India***
~ A woman is polluted and unclean for six week after giving birth. ***Romany Gypsy***
~ Mum is purified by straddling over a pot of herbs on a fire. ***Indonesia***
~ During the first forty days, the new mother is referred to as a 'lehona'. It's bad luck to be visited by a lehona. If she visits your home, you must make her step on a key before she steps in your house to prevent any evil from entering with her. ***Greece***
~ If Mum goes into a strange house; she must first buy something at a strange

place or she brings misfortune to the house. ***Germany*** [1]
~ Mum and Baby aren't allowed to go to Church during the first forty days. After forty days, they must go to church just like the Virgin Mary is said to have done with little Jesus. The priest reads the forty day blessing. If over forty days pass before the blessing is done, then they must wait another forty days before the priest can read the blessing. ***Orthodox Greek***
~ The first time a woman goes to church after a confinement, they throw on the floor after her the pot out of which she has eaten caudle during her six weeks confinement. ***Germany*** [1]
~ Babies up to six months old mustn't come out of the house after twilight. ***India***
~ A baby under one year's old must be kept at home, where he's safe from evil spirits. If Mum absolutely has to take Baby out, she should pierce his ears with gold or red string. (*Philippines)* or Mum and Baby must cover themselves from head to toe. (*Spain*)
~ The mum venturing out for the first time must follow the same path as the sun, if not she'll have a relapse. ***Cornwall UK*** [12]
~ During the confinement and for a short time after the birth, the wife remains in the husband's house, and is then taken to her parents' house where she must live apart from her husband for up to three years. ***West Africa*** [47]

In the first forty days or six weeks, Mum must not:

~ Get on her feet *(Spain)* or get out of bed or do any work for fear of illness. If Mum gives birth to a boy, she should stay in bed a few days longer. (*Japan*)
~ Spin wool, hemp or flax, because the Blessed Virgin did not; else the yarn will be made into a rope for the child to be hanged on some day. ***Germany*** [1]
~ Enter the kitchen (*India),* milk cows, collect eggs, or enter inside a grain store (*Bangladesh.)* or participate in cooking and cleaning, as Mum is considered polluted and polluting. (*Malaysia & Indonesia)*
~ Mum must abstain from the vicinity of a fire and anything that is wooden or earthen. ***Zoroastrian*** [23]
~ Handle dough, as her child's hands will chap. ***Germany*** [1]
~ Mingle with others, perform any religious duty or attend any ceremony, as she's unclean. ***India, Bangladesh & Pakistan***
~ Draw water from a spring, or it will dry up for seven years. If she walks over a garden bed or field she'll make it barren for the next few years, or kill everything. ***Germany*** [1]
~ Sticks pins or needles into curtains as Baby will have bad teeth. ***Germany*** [1]
~ Look at a hill, as it is bad for Mum's menstruation. ***Zoroastrian*** [23]
~ Look out of the window; else every wagon that passes will take a bit of her luck away with it. ***Germany*** [1]
~ As she is vulnerable to evil spirits, Mum is forbidden from leaving the

house. *Malaysia*

BATHING

~ With the bath that she takes within a comparatively few hours after the birth, Mum's isolation, and with it any dangerous influence of her recent condition ceases. *Certain Indian Tribes: Guyana* [21]
~ Mum should not have a bath for several days following birth. *USA*
~ Mum mustn't take cold baths or showers or wash her hair lest she catch cold. *China*
~ A new mum shouldn't wash her head for twenty-one days. *Zoroastrian* [23]
~ Mum must not bathe for three weeks following the birth. *India*
~ For forty days, Mum must not take a shower or bath or wash her hair. Sponge baths, however, are allowed during this period. *Spain*
~ After completion of the couvade, the Grandmother 'smokes' the pathway leading to the water as well as the water itself, before both parents take their first bath. *Tuyuka Indians Guyana* [21]

DRESS CODE

~ If a woman who is confined put a black stomacher on, her child will grow up timid. *Germany* [1]
~ Mum should wear thick clothes to keep warm regardless of season. *China*
~ If Mum goes without new shoes in her first six weeks, her child will have a dangerous fall when he learns to walk. *Germany* [1]
~ Tie a cloth belt firmly around Mum's waist to get her pre-pregnancy figure back quickly. *Philippines*
~ Wrap a sash belt tightly around Mum's waist for four days following birth. *Navajo*

MUM'S DIET

~ Recommended diet for the first four days:
Breakfast: bread and milk, or bread and butter with cocoa
11am: Beef tea and toast
1pm: Poached or boiled egg and milk pudding, or bread and butter
3.30pm: a cup of tea with plenty of milk or cream in it
5.30pm: a cup of cocoa and bread and butter
8.30pm: beef tea, gruel or soup
During the night, a pint of milk or gruel should be taken. On day five, once the bowels have opened, meat may be added. No pickles or acidic fruit should be eaten, and vegetables taken only in moderation. *Edwardian UK* [27]
~ Eating cold food will give fever and cause Mum's womb to swell up. *Thailand*
~ Mum shouldn't eat red meat until her bleeding has stopped. *Native American*
~ Mum shouldn't eat bamboo shoot, eggs or meat, as her stitches will itch and

not heal properly. *Thailand*
~ Mum shouldn't eat squash as it causes fever and dries her up. *China*
~ Mum shouldn't drink cold liquids. *Navajo Tribe: USA*
~ Soon after birth, Mum eats sweet bread. The only fluids she takes are hot chocolate, hot water and chamomile tea. *Guatemala*
~ Mum mustn't eat food considered 'cold'. Mum must eat foods that 'warm' her, the chosen foods also acting as diuretics. The recommended 'warm' foods are ghee, honey, seeds, cassia, cinnamon, comfit, ginger, garlic, clove nutmeg and cardamom. Proteins are to be avoided. Avoiding fluid-based food prevents swelling. *Bangladesh*
~ A special soup made with catfish or pigeon is given to Mum on the third or the seventh day. The mother takes her first cooked rice with this soup. *Bangladesh*
~ Mum should drink juniper tea or ash tea for postpartum cleansing, and drink blue cornmeal mush during her recovery. *Navajo Tribe: USA*

- **MUM'S DIET DURING BREASTFEEDING**

~ Don't eat taro or squash while breastfeeding as it makes Baby itchy. *Philippines*
~ Mum should avoid fish as it makes her milk smell fishy. *Malaysia & Indonesia*
~ Breastfeeding mothers should avoid tomatoes, cabbage and other green vegetables as they give Baby colic. *Romany Gypsy*
~ Mum shouldn't eat 'cool' foods such as melons and cucumbers. *Jewish*
~ The mother should drink beer or whiskey to calm Baby. *Romany Gypsy*
~ Spicy foods cause Baby to be hot-tempered. *Philippines*
~ Nursing mothers should drink a pint of Guinness or Stout a day as it's good for Baby. *1950s UK & Ireland*
~ Marshmallow and red raspberry leaf teas enrich the quality of Mum's breast milk.
~ Should Mum have trouble in producing enough milk, she should: take beef tea or cocoa half an hour before Baby's feed (*Edwardian UK* [27]), drink bitches' milk (*Jewish*) or herbal teas (*India*), eat fennel or honey, take blessed thistle in doses of three cups a day, and apply a poultice of Parsley or take a tablespoonful of brewer's yeast every day.

BREASTFEEDING

~ Colostrum is considered as polluted and too thick for Baby to digest so must be discarded. Baby is fed a mixture of water and gur instead. *India & Pakistan*
~ Before suckling her child, Mum should wipe her breasts three times. *Germany* [1]
~ When Mum nurses Baby for the first time, she must give him her right breast

if she wants him to be right-handed. **Bulgaria, Germany, Holland & USA**
~ If Baby screams after feeding, draws up his legs and has wind and green diarrhoea, then Mum has eaten some indigestible food (the likely cause) or the breast milk is stale. Some breast milk should therefore be drawn off and thrown away before the next feed. **Edwardian UK** [27]
~ Nurse with the left breast first as that's nearer to Mum's heart, the seat of wisdom. **Jewish**
~ When Baby refuses the breast, a Pçuvus-wife (female spirit) must have secretly sucked it. Therefore, place onions between Mum's breasts, and repeat these words:
'*Earth spirit! Earth spirit*
Be thou ill.
Let thy milk be fire
Burn in the earth!
Flow, flow, my milk!
Flow, flow, white milk!
Flow, flow, as I desire
To my hungry child!'
The same incantation is said when milk holds back or won't flow, as it's then supposed a Pçuvus-wife has secretly suckled her own child at Mum's breast. **Romany Gypsy** [7]
~ Mum was encouraged to breastfeed until Baby was three to make her children wise and strong. **Russia**
~ Charm for a Sore Breast to be said in Irish, while a piece of butter is rubbed over the breast. 'O Son, see how swelled is the breast of the woman! O, you that bore a Son, look at it yourself! O Mary! O King of Heaven, let this woman be healed! AMEN.' **Ireland** [15]
~ Mum shouldn't get excited or worry as it detrimentally alters her breast milk, possibly leading to fits in her child. A bottle of boiled cow's milk and water will do the child less harm than the disturbed milk of his mother. **Edwardian UK** [27]
~ If breast milk falls on Baby's penis, he'll become impotent. **Guyana**
~ If Baby's skin is yellow, stop breastfeeding and feed him lots of water instead. **Thailand**
~ After nursing, sponge the nipple with warm boracic lotion, dry and then paint with eau de cologne and glycerine. Wash off solution before the next feed. Nipple cracks can be treated by painting with Tannic Acid in glycerine, and touching occasionally with a piece of blue stone. Again the mixture must be washed off before feeding. **Edwardian UK** [27]
~ If Baby belches on his mother's breast, she should beat his mouth with the breast three times, or the breast will swell and pain her. **Guyana**

The Newborn & New Parents

~ Mum can't get pregnant when breastfeeding. **UK & USA**
~ Extended breastfeeding reduces Baby's intelligence.
~ Cabbage leaves tucked inside Mum's bra provide relief to painful breasts. **UK**
~ If Mum's milk is too rich, give Baby one tablespoon of saccharated limewater before nursing. **Edwardian UK** [27]
~ Breast milk enters Baby's bloodstream, cultivating an unbreakable lifelong spiritual bond with Mum. It also develops character. **Malaysia & Indonesia**
~ Mum helps form the child's spirit while she breastfeeds; her milk is therefore very precious. **Aborigine**
~ A nursing mother (particularly one who does not keep up regular chapel attendance) is at great risk of being abducted by the fairies. The fairies want her to breastfeed their little folk. **Ireland**
~ Smooth breast milk over Baby's eyebrows to make them lush. **Native American**
~ No stranger should enter the house while Baby is still unbaptised, as Mum's milk could dry up. **Germany** [1]
~ Mum shouldn't breastfeed in front of others lest she incurs the 'evil eye' and it poisons her breast milk.
~ Put a piece of animal skin or leather upon the stomach of a breastfeeding baby as an amulet to protect him from harm. **Saudi Arabia**
~ If a woman nurses her baby sitting on the boundary stone at the crossway, he'll never have toothache. **Germany** [1]
~ Mum should never breastfeed within half an hour of sex. **Yugoslavia**
~ Breast milk from a church member cures skin cancer. **USA**
~ If a woman that suckles a boy puts another woman's girl child to her breast, the two children when grown up will come to shame together. **Germany** [1]
~ If Mum's breasts have no milk, her husband fetches the 'tohunga'. When the tohunga arrives, Mum and baby are carried to the waterside, and the tohunga dipping a handful of weed in the water, sprinkles it over Mum. Baby is taken away by the tohunga, who then repeats:
'Water springs from above give me, to pour on the breast of this woman.
Dew of Heaven give me, to cause to trickle the breast of this woman
At the points of the breast of this woman; breasts flowing with milk,
Flowing to the points of the breast of this woman, milk in plenty yielding.
For now the infant cries and moans, in the great night, in the long night.
Tu the benefactor, Tu the giver, Tu the bountiful,
Come to me, to this tauira.'
After this, Baby is dipped in the water, and Mum and Baby are kept apart for one night for the charm to take effect. Mum remains alone in her house, while the tohunga waits outside repeating his charm. Mum is told, 'If the points of

your breasts begin to itch, lay open your clothes, and lie naked.' When her breasts become swollen and painful, Mum calls out for her Baby to be brought back to her. **Maori New Zealand** [48]

~ When two nursing mothers drink at the same time, one drinks the other's milk away. **Germany** [1]

~ Mum must nurse by the clock every two hours between 6am and 10pm for a maximum of fifteen minutes each time. After the baby is one month old, feed by two and a half hour intervals. Irregular feeding is sure to be followed by *evil* consequences. **Edwardian UK** [27]

~ If a baby is breastfed after being weaned, he'll swear constantly when he grows up. **UK & Germany**

~ Don't wind Baby after a meal by rubbing his back, or raising him up, lie him instead on his right side for half an hour so his distended stomach does not press upon his heart. Place Baby in his cradle after each meal, and leave him be so he learns to love his cradle and be content. **Edwardian UK** [27]

~ Rumina is The Roman Goddess of Nursing mothers and Suckling infants

~ Renenet is the Ancient Egyptian Goddess presiding over a baby's suckling.

~ Patron Saints of Nursing Mothers; Concordia, Martina

~ Patron Saint of Breastfeeding: Giles

~ Patron Saint of Loss of Milk by Nursing Mothers: Margaret of Antioch

~ Patron Saints of Wet-nurses: Agatha, Concordia

BOTTLE FEEDING

~ Condensed milk was often given to babies. **UK**

~ Baby is put directly to suckle on the Goat's teat as goat's milk provides immunity to Tuberculosis. **19th Century Europe**

THE NEW FATHER

~ Dad is excluded from Mum's hut for the first eight days from fear he'll be contaminated by the blood of childbirth. He dare not take his baby in his arms for the first three months for this reason. **Bantu Tribe South Africa** [14]

~ Dad won't touch his child until he is several months old for fear that Baby's weakness will cause a corresponding weakness in him. **English Gypsy** [49]

~ A Gallic father, in Caesar's day, would not allow his son to come into his presence until he had grown up and could endure military service. [50]

~ No male can be in the presence of a newborn as long as the cord is attached as it endangers Baby and causes him to follow evil ways. **Loango Tribes Gabon**

~ Dad mustn't see Baby's face until he's six months old as it may cause bad luck. **India**

~ There are various rituals involving the formal recognition of the baby by his father:

Baby is wrapped in swaddling, on which a few drops of paternal blood are

placed,
Baby is covered by a piece of clothing belonging to the father,
Alternatively, Mum puts Baby on the ground and Dad picks him up and places a red string around Baby's neck, thereby acknowledging the child is his. ***Romany Gypsy***

COUVADE

~ After the birth, one or both parents were isolated; in the case of Dad, his 'lying-in' was known as *couvade*, and was practised in many tribes. If the child was a firstborn son, Dad went to bed, complaining and acting as if he'd been delivered himself and submitted himself to a restricted diet. ***Island Carib Indians Guyana*** [21]

~ Straight after the birth, Dad took to his bed and lay groaning with his head tied up, whilst Mum tended him with soup and bread, and prepared his taths. ***The Tiboreni Pontus*** [9]

~ About nineteen hundred years ago, among the Iberians in Northern Spain, the women after the birth tended their husbands, putting them to bed instead of going themselves. This practice still continues among the modern Basques. The women rise immediately after childbirth and attend to the duties of the household, while the husband goes to bed, taking the baby with him, and receives the neighbours' compliments. ***Biscay*** [9]

~ In the thirteenth century, Aucassin arrived at the King of Torelore's palace to find him in couvade. Aucassin took a stick to his majesty, turning him out of bed, while making him promise to abolish this absurd custom in his realm. ***France*** [9]

~ When their wives are confined for the first time, the husband must sling his hammock high up to the ridge of the house and stay there. When the umbilical cord is finally detached, Dad can conclude his 'hatching' or couvade. ***Cayenne Indians*** [21]

~ For ten or twelve days following the birth of his first son, Dad had to take to his bed and eat only cassava and water. After twelve days, he was brought to a public place, where he was whipped and scratched and cut with very sharp agouti teeth or fish bones. The better Dad bore this infliction, the braver his son would be. Dad's blood from the flogging was then smeared on Baby's face to make him courageous. Dad was then painted and rubbed with roucou leaves, pepper seeds and tobacco juice, placed on a red painted seat, and allowed to break his fast. ***Carib Indians Guyana*** [21]

~ Dad's uncleanness was occasionally regarded as persisting for long after the birth. Dad was then obligated to leave his wife for several months and become the slave of an old Indian. ***Carib Indians Guyana*** [21]

~ Dad mustn't bathe during couvade; neither must he scratch himself with his nails. ***Makusi Indians Guyana*** [21]

Baby Lore

~ During the couvade, and often for long afterward, Dad was prohibited from certain occupations. The *Pomeroon Arawak* mustn't smoke, lift heavy weights, use a fishhook, nor have intimate relations with any woman. The *Makusi* must not touch his weapons. Should these and similar prohibitions not be observed, evil would befall the child. There is an example of a man during couvade lying in his hammock and twisting a new bowstring; Baby began to scream, and Dad had to undo the whole line. ***Guyana*** [21]

~ At the end of the couvade, Baby's spirit nature, though *physically* freed from Dad's Spirit, nevertheless accompanies his father until he can crawl. The infant *Spirit* clings to his father, gazes upon him, follows him wherever he goes, and is as intimate and familiar with Dad, as he is with his own infant body with which the Spirit is only recently associated. Dad must therefore be very careful as to what he does, as notwithstanding the greatest vigilance, the little Spirit is sometimes lost, and then Baby's body pines and dies. Therefore, Dad mustn't use an axe, as Baby's infant Spirit which follows Dad as a second shadow might be between the axe and the wood. Dad mustn't climb a tree, as the infant spirit will climb, and perhaps fall, perhaps injuring Baby lying in the hammock at home. Dad mustn't hunt as the arrow might pierce the spirit of the child, which would be death to the little mortal at home. Likewise, anyone travelling through the woods seeing a tairu leaf, which is shaped like a corial boat, floating on water, and furnished with a tiny wooden seat and paddle cut out and placed inside, mustn't disturb it. When Dad wades through the water, the toddling spirit must paddle over in this tairu-leaf boat after him. Anyone discovering two sticks each placed from the ground to the trunk of the tree, should likewise not disturb them as when Dad crosses over the tree stump, the little temporary bridge enables the infant Spirit to climb over after him. ***Indian Tribes Guyana*** [21]

DAD'S DIET

~ If Dad eats turtle, Baby will be heavy and have no brains; if he eats parrot, Baby will have a parrot nose; if he eats crab, Baby will have long legs. ***Carib Indians Guyana*** [21]

~ Dad shouldn't eat red meat until his baby's umbilical cord has fallen off.
Native American

~ Dad must not eat fish or game that has been caught with an arrow; should he disregard this, Baby will soon die or develop vicious tendencies. ***Roucouyenne Indians Guyana*** [21]

CHAPTER 17
DANGERS TO MUM & CHILD

~ If the moon shines on an unbaptised child, he'll be moonstruck. ***Germany*** [1]
~ Gypsies steal children and bring them up because of a superstitious feeling of *bâk*, or luck, and the desire to have a Mascot in the tent. ***Romany Gypsy*** [7]
~ Witches murdered children to secure parts of their bodies for use in their gruesome rites leaving bundles of straw in their place. Witches, midwives in some cases, occasionally removed unborn children by unnatural means from their mothers' wombs and placed them on their altars. ***Ancient Rome*** [51]
~ A child in the cradle who does not look at you is a witch. ***Germany*** [1]
~ A woman on her period can't see a newborn, as she'll 'strain' him. ***Belize***
~ Don't take Baby to a funeral or grave as he has no soul yet. This prevents spirits from getting to him. ***China***
~ A baby under forty days old must not go by a graveyard, or he'll be affected by spirits. ***Turkey***
~ Never take a baby under the age of one year's old to a funeral of a sibling, because if you do, they will die next. ***Portugal***
~ All Baby's problems and sicknesses were explained as evil attack, in the form of spirits, spells or the 'evil eye'. Therefore, the utmost care must be taken to protect the new mother and child from evil influence.

ANIMAL DANGERS

~ The Owl is a bird of ill omen; evil spirits often hide them to carry off children at night. (*Arabia*) Owls bring illness to children (*Swahili*) and their cries can kill babies. (*Morocco*) Owls are also said to eat newborns (*Malaysia*), and in Ancient Rome were thought to be witch-birds that strangled children.
~ Bloodsucking vampires attacked babies in the form of owls. The rites of riddance were as follows: 'Immediately a witch touches the doorposts and threshold three times in succession with arbutus spray. She sprinkles the entrance with water containing a drug. She holds the bloody entrails of a pig, two months old, and says:
 'Birds of the night, spare the entrails of the boy. For a small boy a small victim falls. Take heart for heart, I pray, entrails for entrails. This life we give you in place of a better one.' The witch placed the vital organs in the open air and forbade those attending the rite to look upon them. Then a whitethorn branch was set in a small window. Baby was then safe and the colour returned to his pallid face. ***Ancient Rome*** [52]
~ Cats suck the life out of babies; they steal the baby's breath. ***Europe & USA***
~ During the first seven days, Mum must not strike a cat or she and Baby will

die. *Egypt* [20]

SUPERNATURAL BEINGS

BOGEYMEN – shape-changing spirits who haunt a family and can move objects and cause disruptions. However, a bogeyman can become a playmate for the children. They are vague and formless in appearance, resembling large puffs of dust. A bogeyman can be spotted by quickly looking through a knothole in a wooden partition. If a bogeyman is on the other side, one might catch the dull gleam of his eye before he has time to move away. [26]

JÜDEL OR GÜTEL - the child's lifelong Companion Spirit. Not always bad but can be a nuisance. *Germany*

LAMASTU – a demoness whose principal victims are babies. Miscarriages and cot deaths were attributed to her. She tries to touch the woman's stomach seven times to kill the baby, or kidnaps Baby from nanny. Women wore an amulet of Pazuzu about their necks to protect against her. *Ancient Babylon* [26]

LILITU – a family of demons who haunt the desert and open country. They are especially dangerous to pregnant women and babies. *Ancient Babylon* [26]

LILITH - (a.k.a. 'Baalat' to the Caananites): The fabled first wife of Adam, a bitter demoness out to get new mothers and babies. Lilith's attraction for children is said to come from when God took her demon children away from her when she didn't return to Adam. She therefore launched a reign of terror against women in childbirth and newborns, especially boys. Males were most vulnerable during their first week of life, girls during their first three weeks. *Jewish* [26]

MEJENKWAAR - Often the husband sailed off to collect special items for his pregnant wife. However, if he was gone for too long, Mum could turn into a Mejenkwaad (a type of female demon) and eat her newborn child. When the husband eventually returned, she'd go after him as well. *The Marshall Island: N. Pacific* [26]

THE QARINA - A 'Qarin' or 'Qarina' is the double of an individual, or his familiar demon born at the same time of his birth that is his constant companion throughout life. In the case of males, it's a female mate, and in the case of females, it's a male mate. This evil double is jealous and causes sickness and other problems unless its influence is warded off by magic or religion. *Islamic* [20]

~ When Mum has a boy, her qarin (masculine) has married a qarina (feminine) who gives birth to a girl. This demon child and her mother are jealous of the human mother and child, and seek to harm them. To pacify the jealous qarina, one must sacrifice a completely black chicken. *Egypt* [20]

~ The reason young children die is because Um es Subyan (the child witch) is jealous of the mother, and she uses the child's qarina to kill Baby. Never leave Baby alone for fear of the qarina. Furthermore, the child must not tramp on the ground heavily or he may hurt his qarina and it's dangerous to cast water on the fire lest it vex the qarina. A child's every whim must be satisfied for fear of his evil mate, and on no account must the child be allowed to go asleep while crying. *Egypt* [20]

~ The qarina assume the shape of cats at night; Copts and Moslems dare not hurt a cat after dark for this reason. *Egypt* [20]

SYLVANUS - A god who violently attacks newborns and their mothers. Three protecting divinities, Intercidona, Pilumnus and Deverra were summoned lest Silvanus enter during the night and harass mother and child. *Ancient Rome* [53]

SPRIGGING - ugly, grotesque creatures, who although tiny, can enlarge themselves to the size of giants. Spriggans are clever thieves who steal babies and leave Spriggan babies in their place. [26]

VILA - forest spirits that steal baptised children. *Romany Gypsy* [7]

WILD HUNT & WISH HOUNDS - On the top of the Dewerstone crag, rising above the River Plym, the Wild Huntsman is frequently seen with his fire breathing Wish-hounds. His horn and the yelping of his hounds are heard over the moors as he hunts for human souls.

~ Children who die unbaptised join the hunt. Once two children were on the moor together; one slept, the other was awake. Suddenly the Wild Hunt went by. A voice called, 'Shall we take it?' The answer came, 'No, it will come of itself shortly.' Next day, the sleeper was dead.

~ A farmer was riding over Dartmoor at night when a mysterious hunter with his hounds running before him came up alongside him. The farmer shouted, 'Had good luck; much sport? Give me a hare.' 'Take it,' replied the hunter, and flung something to the farmer. Half an hour later the farmer arrived home, and shouted for a servant to hold his horse. 'Give me the lantern and let me see what I've got.' The farmer, raising the light, saw on his other arm his own child dead. At the same moment it vanished. As he was dismounting, the servant said to him: 'Sorry to have to tell you, farmer, but your poor little boy is dead.' *Devon UK* [9]

~ In Durham, the Wild Hunt goes by the name of the Gabriel Hounds, and in Yorkshire it is called the 'Gabble retchit'.

THE FAIRIES

~ The fairies are the fallen angels, driven out of heaven with Satan. The Manx call them 'Cloan ny moyrn' (the children of the pride). *Ireland & Isle of Man*

~ When God cast the rebellious angels out of heaven, some fell on the mounds or barrows and became Hill folk; others fell into the elf moors and became Elf folk; and others fell into dwellings and became House kobolds. This gives a rough idea of the distinction existing among the 'Little People.' *Jutland: Denmark* [9]

~ Every seven years fairies had to pay 'the teind to hell,' and to save them from paying this tribute with one of themselves, they were ever on the look out for human babies instead. ***Scotland*** [54]

~ The fairies differ from the bugganes and other evil things in that the fairies might be in any place, at any time. ***Isle of Man*** [44]

~ Mab is the Queen of the fairies; a trickster who steals babies.[44]

~ Fairies hide in the drawers and presses to be ready to steal Baby away when he's born, placing some ugly, sickly 'changeling' in the cradle to be brought up by Mum instead. The human child became a servant in the fairy household. Children dying in April are supposed to be carried off by the fairies. ***Ireland*** [15]

~ The Irish are careful not to mention fairies by name either on Wednesdays or Fridays, for these invisible creatures are unusually alert on these two days, and their power for evil is very strong. On Fridays, fairies have the most power to work evil; therefore Friday is an unlucky day to go on a journey, or do anything; for the spirits are then present everywhere, and hear and see everything going on, and will mar and spoil everything they can out of jealousy of the human race. It's then they strike cattle, lame horses, steal milk, and carry away a beautiful mortal child leaving an ugly, wizened little creature in his place. These fairy changelings grow up malicious and wicked, and have voracious appetites without any natural increase in growth. ***Ireland*** [15]

~ Fairies have great power on May Eve, and children must be well guarded from their influence on that day. The Evil Eye also has more than its usual vigilance and malignity then. The nurse (or mother) who walks in the open with a child in her arms on May Eve would be reprobated as a monster. ***Ireland*** [15]

~ The Shetlanders believe in two kinds of trows…those of the land and those of the sea. Termed the 'guid folk' and 'guid neighbours', they live inside green hills. A Shetlander always 'sains' himself (blesses himself) when passing by these hills. The trows have all the thieving inclinations of the Scandinavian trolls and lying-in women and unbaptised babies are regarded as their lawful prize. They employ the mothers as wet nurses, and they rear the babies as their own. Nothing will induce parents to show any attention to a child they suspect of being a 'changeling' but there are parents who undertake to enter the hills and regain their lost child. ***Shetlands Isles Scotland*** [30]

~ The changeling belief was so commonly accepted by many cultures as fact that there's even a Latin treatise, devoted to defining the legal and social status and rights of changelings.[55]

~ A pretty girl must be well guarded or the fairies will carry her off to be

eventually wed to one of their fairy chiefs. ***Ireland***
~ At times, the child has been saved from the fairies as they were carrying him out through the dog-flap. ***Scotland*** [54]
~ Half-fairy children (children of the 'Sidhe') grow up beautiful and clever, but are also wild, reckless and extravagant. They're known at once by the beauty of their eyes and hair, and they have a magic fascination that nobody can resist, specially excelling in music and dancing. They are, however, passionate and wilful, and have strange, moody fits, when they desire solitude above all things, and seem to hold converse with unseen spiritual beings. ***Ireland*** [15]
~ Those people with 'second sight' are probably changelings, or children or grandchildren of changelings that have interbred with humans.
~ Up until at least the 1920s, the disabled were believed to be changelings. The only redress open to parents of a disabled child in the Western Isles of Scotland was to place the imp on the beach below high-water mark, when the tide was out and pay no heed to his screams. It was believed that rather than allow her child to be drowned by the rising waters, the fairy mother would make her appearance, carry it away, and restore the child that had been stolen. [9]
~ When a newborn is knock-kneed, the mother regards him as a changeling. She sits on the threshold on a Tuesday or Friday, when witches are around, and demands the restoration of her own child, whom she believes they have stolen away. 'Give him back you scoundrels!' she exclaims. [3]
~ Even though they were sickly and resembled retards, the changelings could dance and play the fiddle when they thought nobody was looking.
~ A mother believed the piskies put a withered child in her healthy daughter's place. She often saw the pixies come and look over a wall by the house to see the child. And the family once put the child out of doors at night to see if the fairies would take her back again. ***A true story from the Isle of Man***
~ The changeling superstition makes peasant women often very cruel towards weakly children as they test the nature of the suspected 'changeling'. Should there be no improvement in Baby after a concoction of herbs from a 'fairy woman', then the witch sometimes resorts to terrible measures to test the fairy nature of the sufferer. A true story tells of how a child who was suspected of being a change because he was wasted and thin and always restless and fretful was ordered by the witch to be placed for three nights on a shovel outside the door from sunset to sunrise, during which he was given foxglove to chew, and cold water was flung over him to banish the fire devil. The child's screams at night were frightful, calling on his mother to come and take him in; but the fairy doctor told the mother not to fear; the fairies were certainly tormenting him, but by the third night their power would cease, and the child would be restored. However, on the third night, the poor little child lay dead. ***Ireland*** [15]

Baby Lore

~ The trial by fire was often resorted to. The unhappy parents placed Baby in the centre of the cabin, lit a fire round him, and fully expected to see him changed into a sod of turf. But if he survived the ordeal, he was grudgingly accepted as one of the family, and was generally hated by the neighbours for his impish ways. *Ireland* [15]

~ The figure of the cross is made into salt on a shovel. The shovel is placed on the fire near Baby. When the salt gets white-hot, the changeling disappears through the window and the true baby is found unscathed on the doorstep. *Wales*

~ A new skull was hung over the fire from a piece of hazel branch, and the baby was laid into this basket. If Baby screamed, he was a changeling, and he was held fast to prevent his escape. He was then carried to a place where four roads met, and a dead body was carried over him. The true child was then restored. *Scotland* [54]

~ Baby was placed in front of a roaring fire, or was suspended in a basket over the fire. If it was a changeling, it made his escape by the chimney, throwing back words of scorn as it disappeared. *Scotland* [54]

~ Set a pot on the fire and threaten to boil the fairy child, who then vanishes up the chimney and the real child is brought back. *Ireland* [56]

~ To test what the 'squalling, unsightly imp' is, throw it on the fire. 'Seize the child, and throw him into the middle of the fire. If it's your own son you have, he'll call out to save him; but if not, this thing will fly through the roof...' [57]

~ Roast the changeling child upon the live embers, and it will vanish, and the true child will appear where he originally had been taken from. *Scotland* [58]

~ Mum should get a red-hot poker and ram it down her ugly infant's throat. If it be a fairy brat, the fairy mother will come in at the moment and snatch it away. *Ireland*

~ It is far from improbable that there have been many cases of getting rid of babies that did no credit to their mothers; Mum being fully persuaded that the creature she treated in this barbarous manner was really not her own. [9]

~ Less cruel methods of 'testing' a changeling involved brewing 24 empty halves of eggshells in water. Upon seeing this, the changeling will sit up and say with the voice of a very old man; 'What are you doing mammy? I'm fifteen hundred years old and I've seen the egg before the hen. I've seen the first acorn before the oak. But I've never seen brewing in eggshells before!' thus revealing its true old age. Then throw it in the chimney, and the true baby will then be found on the doorstep. *UK*

~ An old woman came into a house and looked at a child without saying 'God bless you'. He got ill, a wise woman told the parents he had been 'changed' and directed them to get a bit of the old woman's cloak. This made the elf sneeze and the true child was brought back. *Ireland* [56]

~ A woman had a child that was remarkably puny. It was greedy enough...but never grew any, and there were shrewd suspicions it was a changeling. One day a neighbour came running into her house, and shouted out, 'Come here, and ye'll see a sight! Yonder's the Fairy Hill a' glowe (on fire).' 'Waes me! what'll come o' my wife and bairns (babies)?' screamed the elf...and straightway made its exit up the chimney. **Scotland** [59]

~ A couple found a baby, and although it looked like a piskie, they cared for it as their own. One day, the grown-up child was looking wistfully out of the house when a voice was heard to call, 'Coleman Gray, Coleman Gray!' The piskie immediately started up, and with a sudden laugh clapped its hands, exclaiming, 'Aha! My daddy is come!' The piskie was gone in a moment, never to be seen again. **Cornwall UK** [12]

~ Fine young peasant women are often carried off by the fairies to breastfeed fairy babies. But the woman is allowed to come back to tend her own infant after sunset. To save her, Dad must throw holy water over her in the name of God at once, and she'll be restored to her own shape. Sometimes she comes with a hissing noise like a serpent; appears black and shrouded like one from the dead; and sometimes, in her own form, when she takes her old place by the fire and nurses her baby; and the husband must ask no questions, but give her food in silence. If she falls asleep the third night, all will be well, then the husband ties a red thread across the door to prevent the fairies coming in to carry her back off, and if the third night passes over safely, the fairies have lost their power over her for ever. **Ireland** [15]

THE EVIL EYE

~ The Evil Eye, called 'Malocchio' in Italian, and 'Mal Ojo' in Spanish, is when someone looks at you or something close to your heart with envy. They may then, intentionally or not, put a hex on you and your family resulting in sickness, injury, poverty, or even death.

~ Those who have the 'evil eye' may not be aware they have it or are doing anything bad.

~ Hairy people, deformed people, and those with a squint or eyebrows that meet in the middle are often thought to be possessors of the evil eye, as also are blue-eyed people in Mediterranean countries.

~ If someone looks enviously at a healthy baby they can 'overlook' him, making him shrink or whither. **Guyana**

~ A baby born with defects means that someone is jealous of the family, and 'overlooked' him or his mother while she was carrying him. **Portugal**

~ A stranger who isn't allowed to cuddle or touch a baby will give the child the evil eye. **Belize**

~ Some mothers wouldn't even let their newborns look at their own fathers for fear of the evil eye. [19]

CHAPTER 18
PROTECTION FROM DANGERS

CHARMS AGAINST THE 'EVIL EYE'

~ If someone in the house is born in January, the house will be safe from the 'evil eye'. *Italy*

~ The colour blue, wards off the evil eye. Blue eye charms made of glass pinned to Baby's clothing or blue bracelets reflect the evil eye back to the person who is unconsciously projecting it. (*Greece & Turkey*) Alternatively, put blue on the sole of Baby's feet (*Belize*)

~ To ward off the evil eye, make the 'mano cornuto' horn sign. This entails making the hand into a fist and extending the index and little finger. This hand gesture has its origins as an ancient amulet. Some children wear a gold 'mano cornuto' charm. *Italy*

~ Alternatively, douse Baby in coconut oil (*Trinidad*), put a piece of coal in Baby's milk (*India*), a spot of soot on Baby's forehead (*Guyana*), or mark a black spot on one side of Baby's forehead and cheek, and tie a black thread around his wrist or to the gold bangles worn on his arm. (*India & Bangladesh*)

~ Hanging a black object on the terrace of a house (*India*), gargoyles (*Europe*), or a metal hand of Fatima over the front door, held up fingers outstretched and pointing towards the evil wisher, also deflects the evil eye (*Egypt* [20])

~ The word 'Garlic' protects from the evil eye. If anyone utters a word of praise with the intention of bewitching or of doing harm, cry aloud 'Garlic!' or utter it three times rapidly. **Poland, Greece & Turkey** [7]

~ Carry a black marble for protection from the 'evil eye' at night, and a white marble for protection during the day. **Bedouin Tribes**

~ A necklace of shells, especially cowries or snail shell, protect children (*Romany Gypsy*), and an Owl's eye worn on a string around the neck is an effective talisman against being 'overlooked'. (*Morocco*)

~ A silver 'Khoumsa' ornament has five points, five being the most powerful of protective agencies. In Moorish folk beliefs, it means the dispersion to the four corners of the earth of any evil influence which has been directed against the wearer. *Morocco*

~ Never take an infant in your arms, nor turn your head to look at him without saying, 'God bless it.' This keeps away the fatal influence of the evil eye. *Ireland*

~ If someone on their period compliments the baby, that person has to touch the baby. If they don't touch the baby, the baby can get 'Ojo' ('eye'). If this happens, say a prayer and crack an egg into a bowl and place it under his crib. Then massage Baby. When the 'ojo' is gone, the egg turns into the shape of an eye. *Spain*

The Newborn & New Parents

~ A couple of dried red chillies are waved over Baby's head and then thrown into the fire. If the smoke doesn't hurt his eyes, it's a sure sign the 'evil eye' has affected him.

~ This is a charm Mary gave to St. Bridget, and she wrote it down and hid it in the hair of her head; 'If a fairy, or a man, or a woman hath overlooked thee, there are three greater in heaven who will cast all evil from thee into the great and terrible sea. Pray to them, and to the seven angels of God, and they'll watch over thee.' ***Ireland*** [15]

~ The evil eye has to be countered by chanting, 'Whoever gave you the evil eye may it fall on them' three times in Yiddish. ***Jewish***

~ The mother of the overlooked child fills her mouth with salt water, and lets it trickle on her infant's limbs, then repeats:
'False (evil) eyes see thee,
Like this water
May they perish
Sickness depart
From thy head,
From thy breast,
From thy belly,
From thy feet
From thy hands,
May they go hence
Into the evil eyes!' ***Romany Gypsy*** [7]

~ A jar is filled with water from a stream that must be taken *with*, not against, the current as it runs. In it are placed seven coals, seven handfuls of meal, and seven cloves of garlic, and this is put on the fire. When the water begins to boil, it's stirred with a three forked twig, while the wise woman repeats:
'Evil eyes look on thee,
May they here extinguished be
And then seven ravens
Pluck out the evil eyes
Evil eyes (now) look on thee.
May they soon extinguished be!
Much dust in the eyes,
Thence may they become blind,
Evil eyes now look on thee;
May they soon extinguished be!
May they burn, May they burn
In the fire of God!' ***Romany Gypsy*** [7]

~ If you think a certain person has caused the 'evil eye', collect a handful of earth on which that person has set foot and circle it thrice clockwise around

Baby's head, and then throw the dirt into the oven. ***India***

Eye henna protection symbol against the 'evil eye'; the cross in the middle deflects evil in four directions. The diamond shape is also protection against the 'evil eye'. The Turkish Nazarlik symbol is very similar to also protect against the 'evil eye'. ***Berber Morocco***
~ Placate the suspected possessor of the evil eye with beer and tobacco. ***Africa***
~ Throw water over the suspected evil eye possessor's footprints.
~ Sick children who are supposed to have been afflicted by the evil eye are washed on the threshold of their cottage, so that with the help of the Penates (guardian spirits) who reside there, the malady may be driven out of doors. ***Lithuania*** [3]

PROTECTIVE CHARMS AGAINST OTHER EVIL

~ The new mother or child must never be left alone. (*Jewish*) A woman who is confined must never be left alone; the devil has more hold upon her then. (*Germany* [1])
~ If a baby is left alone in a room, he'll be changed by the devil for his own. It's believed Albinos are 'changelings'. ***Zanzibar***
~ Parents are careful not to leave Baby alone during his first eight days, within which period the Greek Church refuses to baptise them. Over this period, the newborn must be rocked in his cradle throughout the night to prevent his abduction by evil spirits. ***Greece***
~ Until the mothers were 'sained' and churched and their babies were baptised, the strictest watch had to be kept over them to keep them from being abducted. Women who had been present at the delivery remained in the house for several days to protect the vulnerable mother and child from the 'peerie folk'. For several nights, as many as six women took it in turns to rock the cradle all night so the baby was not stolen away. ***Orkney Isles*** [6]
~ The sixth night is considered a particularly dangerous one, since the evil spirits then become far more active to try to snatch Baby from his mother. Several women stay awake all night, taking it in turns to guard Baby on their laps. ***Muslim Bangladesh***
~ During the first forty days, mothers may not go to sleep until someone else has come to guard the child. ***Germany*** [1]
~ A baby's face should not be powdered with white talcum powder when he is sleeping or his wandering dream spirit will not recognise his face when it's time to be reunited with his body. ***China***

~ Baby's features are painted black so demons will not recognise or desire the infant. A cross is put on his forehead and a spot on his nose. In Selangor, a girl's forehead is marked with a cross, a boy's with a Hindu caste mark. The mother, also, is daubed on her nose and breasts. *Malaysia* [22]
~ Face painting protects the newborn. (*Enkundu-Enkundu Tribe Cameroon*) A black face protects from the evil spirits. (*Bahrein & India*)
~ A child on whom a spell had been cast must be washed in a special preparation of charcoal water. *Romany Gypsy*
~ When a girl is born, lay over her breast a net made of an old (female) cap, and the night elf will not suck her dry. *Germany* [1]
~ An upside-down black kettle placed on a pole, guards the house from evil. *Bahrain*
~ In a lying-in room, lay a straw out of the woman's bed at every door so neither ghost nor Jüdel can get in. *Germany* [1]
~ Keep the nursery door blockaded to prevent dangerous spirits entering. *Europe*
~ All the windows and doors must be kept shut for the first forty nights so the spirit of death called 'the night' can't enter and harm Baby. *Romany Gypsy*
~ The woman of the house must never throw out water after dark without saying: 'Take care of the water,' lest it spoil the fairies colourful caps and feathers and make them angry. *Ireland* [15]
~ Protective little metal hands called 'the hand of Ali' guard Baby. *Iraq*
~ Money, tobacco or beer placed around the nursery placate evil spirits. *Africa*
~ Drive spirits out of the house by beating the furniture with a stick shouting, 'out, out, out, away, away, away, to the red sea, to the red sea, to the red sea,' then clean and lime-wash the house. *Cornwall UK* [12]
~ Three eggs are put in a bowl by Mum's pillow and stay there until she has her ritual postpartum bath. When Mum leaves the house, one egg is broken and thrown out to distract the jinn, another egg when halfway to the bath, and the last egg at the door to the bath, so Mum can enter while the jinn are detained eating. *Iraq* [20]
~ To discover if an infant is bewitched, put under his cradle a vessel full of running water, and drop an egg in; if it floats, the child is bewitched. Or mum should lick Baby's forehead: if bewitched, he'll taste of salt. She should then decontaminate him with sweepings from the four corners of the room with shavings off the four corners of the table with nine sorts of wood. *Germany* [1]
~ To learn whether a child has been 'overlooked' or enchanted, take him to a running stream. Hold Baby's face near to the water, and repeat:
'Water, water, hasten!
Look up, look down
Much water hastens

(May) as much come into the eye
Which looked evil on thee,
And may it now perish.'
If the stream makes a louder sound than usual, then the child is enchanted, but if it runs on as before then something else is the matter. ***Romany Gypsy*** [7]
~ If a child is bewitched, his father should fetch three stalks of straw from different dung heaps and lay them under Baby's pillow. (***Germany*** [1])
Alternately, pull Baby's shirt over his head wrong-side-out and wedge the sleeves or clothes behind the door. (***German Pennsylvania USA***)
~ If a child is fairy struck, give him a cup of cold water in the name of Christ and make the sign of the cross over him. ***Ireland*** [15]
~ If a child does not thrive, he has the Elterlein: shove him a few times into the oven, and the Elterlein is sure to go. If the Jüdel has burnt a child, smear the oven's mouth with bacon rind. ***Germany*** [1]
~ Pinching the possessed child and blowing on his head banishes evil spirits and returns the human spirit to his body. ***Malaysia***
~ Evil spirits can't harm a baby when he's placed inside a magic circle. Spells or diagrams can also be written or drawn inside the circle to add power. ***Jewish & Pagan***
~ A pentagram must be painted on the cradle, or the 'Schlenz' will come and suck the baby dry. ***Germany*** [1]
~ The magic square of Al-Ghazali is hung around children's necks to protect from the 'evil eye' and other evil. Alternately, the magic squares are burnt and Baby is smoked with their fumes; or the squares are hung over the cot. ***Islamic India*** [20]
~ The letters 'AGLA' written in the centre of a hexagram banish evil spirits and misfortune.
~ Care is taken to not mention the good health of the child, lest any human or spirit become jealous and makes Baby ill. ***Vietnam***
~ The 'Holle' Demon that attacks babies is frightened off by tossing Baby into the air three times while shouting Baby's name. ***Germany***
~ Baby photos can't be taken until the eleventh day after birth as Baby doesn't yet have a soul. On the eleventh day, when he's named in a traditional ceremony, Baby receives a soul and can then be photographed. ***India***
~ The newborn is protected from evil spirits by placing a knife, a branch from the echallon tree and other charms beside his head. ***Wolof People Senegal***
~ Relatives of a newborn child do not sleep the first night for fear of the witches. Indeed, a watch is often kept for many nights until the child's baptism. A constant light burns in the room, and an image of a saint is fastened upon the door. A rosary and ravelled napkin are attached to the image, and behind the door a jug of salt and a broom are placed. When a witch comes and sees

the saint's image and the rosary, she usually goes away at once; but even if these talismans are wanting, the salt, napkin, and broom afford adequate protection. For any witch must count the grains of salt, the threads of the napkin's fringe, and the twigs of which the broom is made before entering. And she never has time for all these tasks, because she can't appear before midnight, and must hide herself before dawn. ***Marsala Sicily*** [3]
~ Children's fingers were cut off as the Devil demanded a child's finger to appease his wrath. ***Ancient Greece, Polynesia & Native Americans***
~ After his ritual introduction to earth and water, Baby is laid in a swinging cot made of black cloths hung from a rafter. Into the bunt of the cot are put a cat, a curry-stone, and an iron blade to mislead and terrify evil spirits. ***Malaysia*** [22]
~ Someone not present at the birth must not come in 'on top of the baby' until the first forty days are passed. For this reason, Baby is held over the door so they can enter the room 'under' him. ***Iraq***
~ To ward off sickness and evil spirits, earth from Mohammed's grave is worn in a rag round the child's neck. ***Malaysia***
~ The 'mati' medallion wards off evil spirits and protects Baby from the 'vaskania'. ***Greece***
~ A black bracelet, talisman or image of Buddha ensures Baby's well being. ***China***
~ Amber beads worn as a necklace protect the wearer against illness. ***UK***
~ To protect Baby from witches, put a blue bead somewhere in his clothes.
~ A flat bronze ring three-quarters of an inch in diameter has yellow, red, and blue silk threads tied onto it. It's then hung in the child's armpit to protect against the qarin. ***Egypt***
~ Evil spirits are most powerful at sunset. Children are called indoors and a mother chews 'kuniet terus' (an evil smelling root) supposed to be hated by demons, and spits it out at seven different points as she walks round the house. ***Malaysia*** [20]
~ Infants were made to drink their own urine, and excrement was smeared on babies' nipples to makes them undesirable to evil spirits. ***Slovenia***
~ The Moslem mother often denies the real sex of her baby for seven days after it's born in order to protect its life from the qarina. The 'Seven Covenants of Solomon' is one of the most common amulets against the qarina and/or the child witch. Mum also has verses of the Koran written on the inside of a white dish with musk water or ink. The dish is then filled with water and its contents drunk as a protective charm. ***Egypt***
~ If spiritual attacks have made Baby sickly, Genie's Tongue plant leaves (*Hedyotis congesta*) are infused in his bath. ***Malaysia*** [22]

Baby Lore

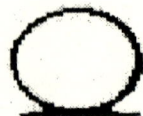
~ Shen Symbol: a loop of rope that has no beginning and no end, symbolising eternity and protection. The sun disk is often depicted in the centre of it. The word shen comes from the word 'shenu', which means 'encircle.' ***Ancient Egypt***

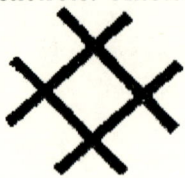
Finger Henna Tattoo Symbol Charm; a protective symbol. ***Berber***

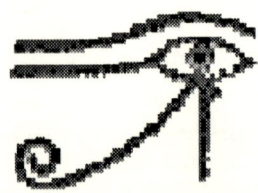
The Eye of Horus ('Udjat') symbolises healing and protection. ***Ancient Egypt***
~ When Baby is mysteriously cranky, has a strange unyielding headache, or can't sleep after a day out, he has been jinxed or exposed to negative energy. Mum should take the lower left corner of her skirt with her right hand and wipe his face several times in a clockwise direction. She should then give Baby some water and put him to bed. ***The Ukraine***

ANIMAL, BIRD & INSECT PROTECTIVE CHARMS
~ Small Lizards protect children and babies. They warn adults if Baby is sick or in danger. ***Native Americans***
~ A wolf's tooth hung around Baby's neck protects against disease. ***Ancient Rome*** [7]
~ The cobra was used as a protective symbol, as the cobra spits fire at approaching enemies. (*Ancient Egypt*) In modern Egypt, every house has a serpent guardian, and many families provide a bowl of milk for their serpent protector, believing it will bring disaster if their serpent is neglected.
~ Animal blood is sprinkled over the doorposts of a sick person's house to ward off the Angel of Death. ***Afghanistan***
~ A chicken's head is hung on the doorframe until after Baby's circumcision. ***Morocco***

~ Hang cockerel's legs over the cradle to protect Baby. *Iraq*
~ Fishtails are hung over doors to guard against evil. *Tunisia*
~ A T-shaped bone from a sheep's head protects from bad luck and evil. To break a curse, stick a sheep's heart full of pins and roast it at midnight in a room where all doors and windows have been firmly closed. *UK*

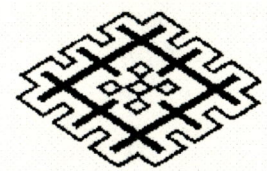 Lion's Paw Henna Symbol: a symbol of strength; the claws are a symbol of protection. *Berber Morocco*

Nose Henna symbol: symbolises the crow's beak worn around a child's neck for protection. *Berber Morocco*
~ The tiger keeps ghosts at bay. *China*
~ A horseshoe picked up from the road and placed over the door will prevent witches from entering the home. *Cornwall UK* [12]
~ The horseshoe over the door or buried under the threshold protects against the Devil, witchcraft, lightning, sickness, and evil of every sort. *Germany* [3]
~ Place a horseshoe with nails in it in the cradle to bring Baby good health. *German Pennsylvania*
~ A horseshoe forged on Saint John's Eve by a bachelor of wholesome life and good character is fixed to the nursery door, lest some rude goblin enters and disturbs Baby's sleep. *Thuringian Forest Germany* [3]
~ Horseshoes hung in the nursery protect against 'nightmares'. *Scandinavia*
~ The reason for the horseshoe's magical power is because the horse and the ass were in the stable where Christ was born, and so became blessed animals. *Ireland* [3]
~ The froth from a horse's mouth repels demons, which fear horses more than any other animal. *Hindustan* [3]
~ Carved wooden horses head's on the gables or placed under the cradle safeguard from demons and sickness. *Germany* [3]
~ A horse's skull placed over a courtyard gate protects against ghosts. *Romania* [3]
~ Dried donkey tongue is a powerful charm against the qarina. *Egypt*
~ Put Baby to sleep on donkey skin to keep away devils and ghosts.

BELLS
~ The sound of bells drives away demons, witches and fairies because they're

afraid of the loud noise. Bells also drive off the plague and other sicknesses. (*Europe*) On a Friday, the church bells strike the hour for the release of bewitched spirits, and the delivery of enchanted souls from their spells. [3]
~ Silver or horn baby rattles with tiny bells protect Baby from fairy abduction (*Scotland*) and bells hung on the cradle guard against demons. (*Jewish*)
~ When a child gradually wastes away, the mother concludes a demon has entered her child. To lure the demon out, she offers a sacrifice of food; and while the devil is eating it, she attaches iron rings and bells to her child's ankles and hangs iron chains around his neck. The jingling of the iron and the tinkling of the bells prevent the demon, when he has finished his meal, from re-entering Baby's body. ***Africa Slave Coast*** [14]

BROOMS

~ Baby can't be left alone at any time; if it becomes absolutely necessary, then a broom is placed beside him. ***Turkey***
~ A broom laid beneath the child's pillow will keep spirits away. ***Tuscany*** [7]
~ If Mum is pestered by visitors whom she wishes never to see again, she should sprinkle salt on the floor and sweep it out by the same door through which they have left, and they'll never return. ***Creole USA***
~ If bewitched, lay a broom by the door. The 'rules' decree, the first person to come in and pick up the broom is the witch. ***German Pennsylvania USA***

CLOTHES

~ Victims of occult attack should wear their shoes on the wrong feet, and their clothes inside-out. ***Voodoo***
~ Every time Mum leaves the room, let her spread some garment of the father's over the child, and he cannot then be a changeling. (*Germany* [1])The father's trousers put across the child are considered a good preservative against the fairies. (*Isle of Man*[44])
~ 'The little one's safeguard lies in the use of some clothing belonging to his father. This was experienced by a shepherd's wife from near Selkirk. Soon after the birth of her first child, a fine boy, she was lying in bed with her baby by her side, when suddenly she became aware of a confused noise of talking and laughter in the room. This proceeded from the fairies, who were forming a child of wax as a substitute for her baby, whom they were planning to steal away. The poor mother suspected as much, so in great alarm she seized her husband's waistcoat, which chanced to be lying at the foot of the bed, and flung it over herself and the child. The fairies set up a loud scream, calling out, 'Auld Luckie has cheated us o' our bairnie!' Soon afterwards, the woman heard something fall down the chimney, and looking out she saw a waxen image of her baby, stuck full of pins, lying on the hearth. When her husband came home, he made up a large fire and threw the fairy lump upon it; but, instead of burning, `the thing flew up the chimney, and the house instantly

resounded with shouts of joy and peals of laughter.' **Scotland** [60]

DEALING WITH COMPLIMENTS

~ If anyone compliments Baby, someone must say, 'God bless' to immediately ward off evil spirits. (*Portugal, Brazil & Ireland*) Never praise Baby aloud without first saying 'God save it' or 'Safe be it'. Without these precautions, the child is said to be 'forespoken,' confirming that Baby is almost too good to live. (*Orkney Isles* [6])

~ Never say good words about a baby, evil spirits will hear them and may want to harm Baby as a result. *(Kyrgyzstan)* Never say Baby is beautiful, or the Ghost Mother will take him away. (*Thailand*)

~ Praise should never be given to a newborn as this invites the attention of demons and ghosts who may steal the child because of his desirability. Baby should therefore be referred to with unfavourable words. *(China & Vietnam)* Greet newborns with expressions such as, 'you are ugly,' to protect them (*Hmong People Asia*) If someone praises Baby, Mum should always say something derogatory about her child to compensate. (*Asia*)

~ Whenever someone compliments her baby, Mum should knock on unpolished wood or spit three times over her left shoulder to chase off evil. **Russia**

~ Complimenting a baby means he might turn out the opposite. Therefore babies must to be ridiculed so they don't turn out ugly. **Hmong People Asia**

~ Those who admire a baby must touch him with their hand to show the absence of envy. **Mexico**

~ If you see a baby and think he's cute, you must pinch him, or you'll steal his soul and he'll get sick. **The Chamorro: Guam**

FIRE & LIGHT

~ Placate the fairies by keeping them warm at night, and they will cause you and your baby no harm. (*Western Isles of Scotland*) The fairies like people who are kind and considerate, and who leave food on the dresser and fire in the grate at night for when they hold their councils; yet not too much fire, for they dislike smoke. (*Ireland* [15])

~ Bonfires and other light sources drive away malevolent spirits. It was traditional to build fires at Midsummer, Halloween, and Lammas, when the spirits were said to be at their most potent. On Halloween, when danger from evil peaks, turnips with candles inside (jack-o'-lanterns) protect from evil. The lanterns were placed around the house, especially within Baby's room. (*UK*)

~ In old times, at Whitsuntide (considered a dangerous time), children and cattle were passed through two lines of fire. **Ireland** [15]

~ Just after Baby's birth, a fire is lit to drive evil spirits away. Both Muslim and Hindu families also keep a lamp burning throughout the night for seven days. **Bangladesh**

~ A fire is kept up until Baby is baptised to ban the devil, and keep him from 'changing' the child. ***Estonia***[1]
~ Burn a lamp or fire for Baby's first three nights and days so the demons and fiends may not be able to do him any harm. According to scripture, every night, for three nights, a demon came with a hundred and fifty other demons, to slaughter Zartosht, and when they saw the light of the fire, they fled away, and were not able to do him any harm. ***Zoroastrion*** [23]
~ Candles near the beds drive away spirits. ***Medieval Europe***
~ Candles are lit on the seventh day and placed in a jug of water near the head of the baby, to guard him against the qarina. ***Egypt***
~ Baby is kept carefully concealed within thick curtains, while a smoking light is kept burning within the curtains day and night. Baby is also surrounded by large squares of paper with flaming hands and outspread fingers. ***Jewish***
~ Light and/or fire is a great safeguard against evil, especially when someone is sick, for evil spirits are then on the lookout to carry off victims. ***Ireland*** [15]
~ On Wednesdays and Fridays (when the fairies are particularly evil) a careful watch is kept over the children; a lighted wisp of straw is waved about Baby's head, and a quenched spent red coal is placed underneath his cradle. ***Ireland*** [3]

FLOWERS, HERBS & TREES

~ Rowan and St. John's Wort hung over the doorway stops evil spirits from entering. ***UK***
~ A branch of the rowan tree was placed over a door, after being waved around while chanting the words, 'Avaunt, Satan!' ***Northern Scotland*** [3]
~ Rosemary planted by the door keeps witches away. ***UK***
~ Scatter primroses before the door, for the fairies can't pass the flowers. ***Ireland*** [15]
~ Magic qualities are attached to the lime or linden tree; in some villages it is usual to plant one before a house to prevent witches from entering. ***Hungary & Germany***
~ Hawthorn hedges were planted as protective spiritual shields around houses. ***Celtic***
~ A branch of aloe protects against objectionable spiritual intruders. ***Egypt***
~ An oak front door, and an oak door to the nursery protects against evil from entering. A cradle made from oak is excellent because of the oak tree's spiritual guardian powers. ***Celtic***
~ Mum should put flowers under Baby's cot to placate the fairies.
~ Rowan and mistletoe tied to the cradle protects Baby from fairy abduction
~ A bowl of primroses under the cradle offers protection against witches.
~ Clover protects babies from witch's spells and fairies, and brings good luck.
~ Angelica and nettle worn as an amulet will protect Baby from evil spirits.
~ Lay snapdragon, blue marjoram, black cumin, a right shirtsleeve, and a left

stocking into the cradle. The 'Nickert' cannot then harm the child. ***Germany*** [1]
~ Place an anemone flower near Baby or a pine branch over his bed to keep illness away. ***UK***
~ Bathing Baby in fennel water protects him against the spirit of disease. ***UK***
~ A bundle of twigs from the oak, ash and thorn, tied together and placed in the nursery, will protect against fairies. ***Ireland***
~ The ash tree's branches or twigs stops snakes approaching children. ***Cornwall: UK***
~ A branch of mountain ash tied over the cradle protects girls against fairy abduction, as according to ancient superstition the first woman was created from the mountain ash. A branch of the alder tree protects boys, as the first man was created from an alder tree. ***Ireland***
~ Place lilacs around the house to rid yourself of unwanted spirits. ***Pagan***
~ Sage has strong protective powers. ***Southern Europe***
~ Plant houseleeks on the roof to stop ghosts entering. The Latin name for this plant, 'sempervivium', means 'ever living' and the dead can't stand its presence.

FOOD

~ Always leave food out for the fairies so they don't become angry and curse the home. Any food left out overnight is fairy food and shouldn't be eaten by the family as it's taking it away from the fairies. ***Ireland***
~ Put sweets under the bed of a new mother to occupy evil spirits and keep them away from Baby. ***Yemeni Jews***
~ At dusk, leave out dishes of food and keep bread under the cot or cot mattress to appease the jinn. ***Egypt & Morocco***
~ If taking Baby anywhere at night, always take along a piece of bread so if the fairies are around they'll take the bread and not the child. ***Newfoundland***
~ Garlic magically protects against poison and sorcery. According to Pliny, this is because when it's hung up in the open air for a time, it turns black. It's thus believed to be attracting evil into itself away from the wearer. ***Ancient Rome*** [7]
~ During the dangerous forty days period, garlic amulets should be worn by Mum and Baby to ward off evil spirits. ***Somalia***
~ Guard against evil spirits by placing in the cradle or over the door, garlic slat bread. (***Denmark***), or lay garlic under Baby's pillow. (***Poland*** [7])
~ Garlic hung in a corner of the house wards off vampires, witches, spirits and the evil eye. ***Southern & Eastern Europe***
~ The magic virtues of garlic are also attributed to onion and leek.
~ Scatter some salt or sugar around to purify a room. ***Pagan***
~ A newborn should swallow fresh butter to protect him from the fairies. ***Scotland***

~ Put a large apple beneath a child's pillow on Halloween to protect him from spirits. **Cornwall UK**
~ Eggshells are favourite havens of the fairies; therefore always break up the eggshell after use to prevent a fairy taking up home there. **Ireland**
~ An egg built into a new building protects it against evil and witchcraft. **Germany** [7]
~ Evil spirits will not enter a house in which there is a citron. **Islamic** [20]
~ Before the child is born, a special amulet is prepared, consisting of seven grains each of seven different kinds of cereal. These are sewn up in a bag, for Baby to wear continuously to guard against the qarina. **Egypt**

IRON

~ Placing a knife on the doorstep will prevent harm entering the house. A knife placed in the cradle protects the helpless newborn against fairies. **Scotland**
~ Hang a carving knife from the head of the cradle with the point suspended near Baby's face. **West Yorkshire UK**
~ In the cradle, hide a sword or knife with its point sticking out: if evil tries to get over mother or child, it will fall upon it. **Germany** [1]
~ Under Mum's pillow or mattress is laid a knife, without which Mum may never leave her bed. **Jewish**
~ Moroccan iron is considered a great protection against demons; hence it's usual to place a knife or dagger under a sick child's pillow.
'Let the superstitious wife
Near the child's heart lay a knife,
Point be up, and haft be down;
While she gossips in the town.
This 'mong other mystic charms
Keeps the sleeping child from harms' **UK** [5]
~ A dagger is stuck in the ground near Mum's head; and every day for thirty days it's carried around Mum's bed three times to guard against the werewolf and the wicked fairies. While taking the dagger around the bed they sing; 'I make a circle, as many tiles as are on this roof, so many angels keep watch over us!' **German Jewish**
~ Mum and her children should wear iron anklets to ward off the qarin. **Egypt**.
~ A pair of scissors should be carried around at all times by Mum to protect evil from coming near. (*Indonesia*) A pair of shears also protects from evil. (*Italy*)
~ Put a pair of scissors under Baby's pillow to keep off evil spirits. **Guyana**
~ Place in the cradle, or over the door, iron or steel in the form of some sharp instrument. **Denmark**
~ The first time Baby is laid in the cradle, they put a knife, a cross key, and

some red yarn beside him to defend from sorcery. ***Estonia***[1]

Scissors Protection Henna Symbol: a symbol of metalworkers, whose occupation is treated with fearful respect as metal keeps away the Jinn. ***Berber***
~ A piece of iron should be hidden beneath the crib so the fairies will be unable to steal Baby away *(UK)* or should be sewn into Baby's clothes, and kept there until after the baptism. (*Ireland*)
~ Nails in the front of a bed or cot ward off the fairies from new mothers and babies.
~ A piece of iron in a breastfeeding woman's pocket is enough to prevent the fairies abducting her at night.
~ Put a key beside Baby so he can't be taken for a changeling. ***Germany & Italy***

The Troll Cross is a powerful protective symbol, efficient on both evil trolls and other similar beings that might be lurking in the woods. Iron and steel is feared by the trolls, and steel in a crosswise pattern makes the charm even more efficient. ***Scandinavia*** [8]
~ Lodestone is a protective talisman against spirits. This may be due to its association with iron.

MIRRORS
~ Although fairies love to look at their reflections in pools of water, they hate mirrors. Hanging up mirrors near the home's entrance will guard against the fairies. Some even put a tiny mirror within the cot for the same reason.
~ Mirrors are placed on front doors. If a dragon tries to get in, he'll see his reflection, think there is already a dragon there, and go away. ***Vietnam***
~ A Mirror of any size placed opposite the front door will reflect back out of the door any evil or spell that comes in.

NAMING BABY
~ In many cultures, knowing the name of something or somebody gives you power over it. If you don't know the name, you're powerless. Therefore, mothers make great efforts to conceal their baby's real names so evil can't reach them.

~ An enemy, who knows your name, has in it something he can use magically to your detriment. ***Aborigine***[14]

~ A name isn't just a mere label, but a distinct part of someone's personality. The malicious handling of a name brings as much injury as a physical wound. ***Native American***

~ If you write a person's name down you can carry off his soul along with it. ***The Tolampoos of Celebes Indonesia***[14]

~ Keep Baby's name a secret and don't utter it aloud; for there are fairies or imps who, if they know Baby's name, will do him an injury; but as long as these fairies don't know his name, they're powerless. ***Chiloe Island Chile***[14]

~ Baby's names are never spoken, so demons can't assault them as a result of hearing their true names. ***Nias North Sumatra***[14]

~ Besides a personal name which is in common use, the older men give Baby a secret name soon after birth which is known only to the fully initiated. This secret name is never mentioned except upon the most solemn occasions; to utter it in the hearing of another group is a most serious breach of tribal custom. When mentioned at all, the name is spoken only in a whisper, and not until the most elaborate precautions have been taken. ***Aborigine: Australia***[14]

~ Every Egyptian received two names, the 'true' name and the 'good' name, or the 'great' name and the 'little' name; and while the good or little name was made public, the true or great name was carefully concealed. ***Ancient Egypt***[14]

~ A Brahman child receives two names, one for common use, and the other that only his father and mother know. The secret name is only used at ceremonies such as marriage, and is intended to protect the child against magic, since a charm is only effective in combination with the real name. ***India***

~ The 'milk name' is a nickname used until the child starts school, or even up until marriage. If given a milk name, a girl's name will often be chosen for a boy, because it's thought a boy is especially coveted by evil spirits and these spirits will be tricked if the boy has a girl's name. A girl is usually given an animal name as protection. ***China***

~ The Angel of Death could inadvertently look over a baby with the name of one already dead. A baby born after a previous cot death is called 'Alter' for boys or 'Alte' for girls, meaning 'the old one,' in the hope the Angel of Death is fooled. The child receives a new name only after reaching maturity. ***German Jews***[2]

~ When the first two children die, the death of the third child is averted by giving the child a humble name like Kuppusamy (Lord of Refuse), Kuppammal (Lady of Refuse), Pakri (Fakir) or Pichai (Beggar). They also disfigure Baby's face, by piercing his left nostril and putting a gold wire ring through it. These mutilations make the child ugly and thus undesirable from

the evil spirits causing death. *India*
~ The medicine men not only gave names to the children, but also under certain circumstances change them. After treating a sick child, the 'Pia' may give Baby a new name, thus enabling him to make a fresh start. ***Arawak Indians Guyana*** [21]
~ Illness is the work of some spiteful demon. Therefore, when Baby recovers, his name should be changed so the demon may not recognise him again. ***Native Americans*** [3]
~ The mere mention of unpleasant names suffices to frighten away the demons who cause sickness; these spirits are also deceived by simply changing the name of a sick child. ***West Africa*** [3]
~ Hateful names given to ailing children are thought to terrify the evil spirits; but when the little patients recover, pleasanter names are substituted. ***Tonquin Southeast Asia***
~ If you want children to live long, call the boys Adam, and the girls Eve. ***Europe***

RED ITEMS

~ A Red Ribbon has kabbalistic powers of protection. Put a red ribbon on the cradle to keep evil spirits away. ***Jewish***
~ To protect from spells and curses that could change Baby into an ugly child, a red ribbon is tied to his wrist. (*Romany Gypsy*)
~ Tie a red ribbon around Baby's wrist so nobody can 'overlook' him. (*Belize, Slavic, Holland & Germany*) Wearing a hidden ribbon is more potent. (*Italy*)
~ If a child has recently been ill, a red ribbon will prevent the illness from returning.
~ Tie a red thread across the door to prevent the fairies entering. ***Ireland***
~ Blood and anything that looks like blood has the power to drive away evil. Emperor Albinus's family (196 A.D) had their newborns wrapped in bandages of a reddish colour for this reason. ***Ancient Rome*** [16]
~ Dress your little girl in red, or at the least put a red ribbon in her hair, to protect her from evil.

SALT

~ Salt has long enjoyed a reputation as a means of procuring disenchantment. It was an ingredient of a salve 'against nocturnal goblin visitors' used by the Anglo-Saxons, while in the annals of folk medicine are to be found numerous references to its reputed virtues as a magical therapeutic agent. In Scotland, when a person is ailing of some affection whose nature is not apparent, as much salt as can be placed on a sixpence is dissolved in water, and the solution is then applied three times to the soles of the patient's feet, to the palms of his hands, and to his forehead. He is then expected to taste the mixture, a portion of which is thrown over the fire while saying, 'Lord,

preserve us frae a' skaith.' [3]
~ Mix salt and pepper together and scatter it around the house to dispel evil. ***Pagan***
~ The best protection from fairies is a little salt tied up in Baby's clothes when he is put to sleep in his cradle. ***Ireland***
~ To protect against demons, place a handful of salt in the cradle (*Jewish*), a plate of salt on the child (*Italy*), or rub Baby in salt. (*Jewish & Slavic*)
~ Before the child is baptised, Mum puts Baby in a casket, and places by his side salt and candles. This custom is expressed in the ancient ballad entitled 'The King's Daughter';
*'The bairnie she swyl'd in linen so fine,
In a gilded casket she laid it syne,
Mickle saut and light she laid therein,
Cause yet in God's house it had'na been.'* ***Scotland*** [3]

SPITTING

~ To avert the evil eye, relatives spat on Baby saying, 'aren't you ugly' (*Slovenia*), spittle was applied to Baby's forehead and lips with the middle finger (*Ancient Rome*), and they tied a thread of diverse colours about Baby's neck then spat on the ground, and mixing the spittle with dirt, put it upon Baby's forehead and lips.[19]
~ After admiring a baby, you must spit to avoid accidentally giving him the 'evil eye' (*Italy*), the person who compliments a baby should spit three times on the baby for luck (*Asia*), or grandma spits three times, 'Pooh, pooh, pooh.' to ward off evil. (*Jewish*)
~ Old women averted the evil eye from babies by spitting into their bosoms three times; three being a sacred number.
~ When anyone looked upon a sleeping baby, it was usual for the nurse to spit three times upon the ground. She did this, even though infants are under the especial guardianship of the god Fascinus, the protector also of generals. Fascinus's image is attached beneath the triumphal car, to protect the victorious general against the effects of envy. ***Ancient Rome*** [16]
~ Spit three times in the face of the overlooked to break the spell. ***Ancient Greece*** [15]
~ Burn a piece cut from Baby's dress to a tinder and grind to a powder which Baby must drink, then anointing his forehead with spittle three times. [15]
~ A newborn must be spat on to secure his health and preservation. ***Bahrain***
~ Spitting chases the devil and bad luck away. That's why when someone talks about bad news, the others spit three time saying 'ftou, ftou, ftou'. ***Greece***
~ Spit on the hands to ward off evil spirits. ***South Africa***
~ A 'taleb' will spit in the mouth of a patient possessed by 'jinn', knocking him sharply on the back between the shoulder blades, and the evil spirit will

leave him. ***Algeria*** [20]

~ The spit is 'soul stuff' that can transfer good and can be used for curing sickness. Arab women stand outside the entrance to the mosque with cups in their hands. They wait to collect the spit of the men who are coming out after prayers, to use on their sick ones at home. Some spit on bread and salt instead, to be fed to the sick. ***Islamic*** [20]

~ Saliva mixed with oil is used as an ointment and is also taken internally. It's collected in a cup from various contributors. ***Bahrain*** [20]

~ Someone spits on his hands and wipes them over a sick baby's face and hands. ***Tunisia***

CHAPTER 19
RELIGIOUS PROTECTION

~ Going to church regularly offers good protection from every evil. *Europe*
~ Wear a gospel around the neck, and keep an errub and a bit of a burnt sod from St. John's Night sewn up in the clothes to guard against fairy abduction. *Ireland*
~ An open Bible is placed somewhere in the room. *Italy*
~ No evil spirit visits the room where a holy book lies in a place of honour; that is the highest shelf. *Islamic*
~ The Bible is placed under the cradle. Some believe it has to be hidden to be effective. *Orkney Islands*
~ Put a bible (*Guyana*), a copy of the Koran tied up in a scarf (*Iraq*), any holy book (*Rumanian Jews*), hidden amulets written with Holy Scripture (*Jewish & Islamic*) or a hymnbook (*Estonia*[1]) under Baby's pillow for luck and to keep off the spirits.
~ Passages from the Koran are painted as murals on the walls to ward off the evil eye. *Islamic*
~ Put sacred words on the doorposts and holy oil above the lintel. *Jewish*
~ Religious exhortations are placed over the entrances such as, 'This house is in God's hand; May Good Luck come in, and Bad Luck stay out!' And 'All persons entering this house are recommended to Divine protection. God and the Virgin Mary guard all such, even though powerful enemies threaten, and lightening and thunder rage without!' *Germany & Austria* [3]
~ The rosary is used to protect against the 'evil eye', sickness and other dangers. *Islamic Countries*
~ Protect homes with the displaying of a 'Himmelsbrief' letter of protection. *Germany*
~ A crucifix or cross and holy water guard the home. Anoint Baby's head or the rest of the room with oil in the sign of cross. The name of Jesus drives away all sicknesses and evil spirits. *Christian*
~ Sacred water combined with incense expels the grasshopper demon. *Malaysia*
~ During Baby's first thirty days, schoolchildren recite evening prayers in the lying-in chamber, in order to keep off the elves. *Jewish*

PROTECTIVE GODS & GODDESSES

Balit-il: Babylonian protector of newborns
Cunina: Roman Guardian goddess of the cradle. In addition to having the power to avert the evil eye, she supplied quiet.
Pihsia yuan chein: Chinese protector of mothers and children

Jizo Bosatsu: Japanese protector of the young
Levana: presided over the ceremonial lifting of the child from the ground by the father. It has been suggested that the newborn was placed on the ground so he might receive a soul from Mother Earth; as babies at birth don't have souls. *Ancient Rome* [16]
Syen: Slavonic guardian spirits of the home

ROMAN CATHOLIC PATRON SAINTS

Patron Saints of newborn babies & infants: Brigid of Ireland, Holy Innocents, Nicholas of Tolentino, Philip of Zell, Philomena, Raymond Nonnatus, Zeno of Verona

Patron Saint of Children: Bathild, Gabriel Gowdel, Gerard Majella, Infant Jesus of Prague, Maria Goretti, Nicholas of Myra, Pancras, Philomena, Raymond Nonnatus, Solange, Symphorian of Autun, Trophimus of Arles

Patron Saint of Illegitimate Children: Brigid of Ireland, Eustochium of Padua, Sibyllina Biscossi

Patron Saints of Mothers: Anne, Gerard Majella, Monica

Patron Saints of Fathers: Joachim, Joseph

Patron Saints against Evil Spirits: Agrippina, Demetrius of Sermium, Quirinus

BAPTISM

~ The child's baptism is his ultimate protection from evil spirits and fairy abduction.

~ John the Baptist is the Patron Saint of baptism. *Roman Catholic*

BELIEFS REGARDING UNBAPTISED BABIES

~ It's unlucky to bring an unbaptised child into the house. *UK*

~ It's not safe to take an unbaptised child in your arms without making the sign of the cross over it. *Ireland*

~ It's unlucky to give a coal of fire out of the house before Baby is baptised. *Ireland*

~ A baby left unbaptised long gets fine large eyes. *Germany* [1]

~ Children dying unbaptised turn into butterflies (*Germany)*, become pixies (*Devon*) do nothing but sit upon fairy stools (*Ireland),* join the phantom Wish or Yeth Hounds that eternally hunt across Dartmoor (*Devon*) or join the Furious Host. (*Germany* [1])

~ An unbaptised baby can't go to heaven. *Most Catholic countries*

~ An unbaptised baby will not attain to the same joy in heaven that a baptised child does and is doomed to carry a perpetual light resembling a candle. *Isle of Man* [44]

~ The peasantry believed the stars were human souls. When a child died, his spirit was taken up to heaven and hung there as a star, but unbaptised children's souls became willo-the-wisps. ***Germany***[9]

~ An Eary Cushlin heiress was an unmarried mother, and to hide her shame her baby was 'done away with' without being baptised. And every night as the fishermen were out fishing they heard a child crying on the shore. One night a fisherman asked why it was crying, when he received the answer: 'I'm a little child without a name.' Then the man shouted back: 'If you are a girl I name you Joney, and if you are a boy I name you John.' After that the crying ceased and the child was heard no more. *Isle of Man*[44]

~ In Northern England, people avoided stepping over the graves of unbaptised children, but in Wales and the South, these graves were considered lucky.

~ Unborn children are luminous, and this has resulted in many murders of pregnant women, by men who desired to get hold of a hand of an unborn, unbaptised child, to use as a charm to send all who live in a house to sleep so they could rob it.[9]

BAPTISM CEREMONY

~ In choosing godparents, ask an unmarried woman, or the child will be unlucky in marriage, and have no children. ***Germany***[1]

~ If a bachelor and spinster stand sponsors to a child, the priest shall stand between the two, or they'll always be falling out. ***Germany***[1]

~ If a child is to live one hundred years, the godparents must be fetched from three parishes. ***Germany***[1]

~ A pregnant woman isn't allowed to be a godmother as Baby will have bad luck. (*Scotland*) or the baby she's carrying, or the child being baptised, will die. (*Ireland*)

~ A child shouldn't be baptised on another child's birthday or directly after a burial, or the child will follow the dead. Baptism has most power on a Thursday. *Estonia*[1]

~ If the baptism is on a Wednesday or Friday (*Germany*) or a Friday (*Estonia*), Baby will grow up a rogue, and go to the gallows.[1]

~ A baby girl was baptised and confirmed as early as possible to bring about an early marriage for her. *Russia*

~ Tying rings to the swathings of a baptised boy, makes him marry early. *Estonia*[1]

~ Salt was carried around the unbaptised child 'withershins' (backwards) to protect Baby from evil during the sometimes long journey to the church where the ceremony was to be performed. *Scotland*[3]

~ A piece of bread and cheese were placed in Baby's clothing to guard against fairy abduction en-route to the Church. *Ireland*

~ In Baby's clothes, some insert money, bread, and garlic; then the first two will never fail him, and garlic protects from sorcery.

~ Some babies wear a 'filakto' which is a small cloth pouch containing something religious such as a flower from the Epitaphio, a little piece of the holy cross, or some soil from Jerusalem. This is pinned on Baby's left shoulder blade. *Greek Orthodox*

~ Mum should put her clothing on inside-out and tuck a piece of garlic and bread inside to protect her from the 'evil eye' at the Baptism. *Russia*

~ Mum should wear new shoes, or her child will have a bad fall when he learns to run alone. *Germany* [1]

~ The godparents should borrow something to wear, so Baby will always have credit. If they put clean clothes on, no witch can get at the child. *Germany* [1]

~ A godparent shall not go to toilet after he is dressed for church; else his godchild will wet the bed. *France*

~ A godparent mustn't eat meat just before the service, as he'll give Baby toothache. *Estonia*[1]

~ Before leaving for the service, Mum should stride over a broom. *Germany* [1]

~ Those that have lost children before shouldn't take Baby out by the door, but should pass him out through the window instead. Baby will be the stronger, and live the longer as a result. *Germany* [1]

~ Give the first person you meet on the way to the baptism a piece of bread with salt for luck. 'Kimbly' is the name of a piece of bread or cake given in rural areas to the first person met when going to a christening. *Cornwall UK* [12]

~ If a living worm is put into Baby's hand before he's baptised, and kept there until the worm is dead, then Baby gains power to cure all childhood diseases. *Ireland* [15]

~ The first child christened at a newly consecrated font receives the gift of seeing spirits and things to come until someone out of curiosity steps on his left foot and looks over his right shoulder; then the gift passes to him. But that can be prevented by the sponsors dropping a straw, a pin or a piece of paper into the basin. *Germany* [1]

~ A child baptised in a new font in a new church becomes the Devil's. *Yorkshire* [9]

~ When none but girls are brought to the font, they will go unmarried for a long time, perhaps forever. *Estonia* [1]

~ Where several children are to be baptised at the same time, a girl mustn't be baptised before a boy as she will acquire a beard and moustache, and the boy will grow up smooth faced. *Yorkshire, Durham & Orkney Isles* [9]

~ The Holy Well at St Ludgvan was celebrated, for every child baptised in its waters would be free from the hangman's rope. As one could be hanged for thieving, this water was very much in demand by the peasantry from far and wide. *Cornwall UK* [12]

~ If three drops of water are given to Baby before he's baptised, he'll answer the first three questions put to him. *Ireland* [15]

Baby Lore

~ Leave Baby's hands free so he'll be quick and industrious. ***Estonia*** [1]

~ During the service, godparents shouldn't look around or the child will see ghosts, and nobody must talk, or Baby will talk in his sleep. ***Estonia*** [1]

~ It's very important to progress in all matters from left to right, or in the path of the sun. A number of children were brought to be baptised, and were ranged in a group around the font. The officiating minister, however, began with the child on his *right* hand, going around to the child on his left. This action caused great indignation: some parents were quite sure that their children had not been done properly and felt they must be taken to another church 'to be done over again.' Likewise, it's most unlucky to be on the left side of the bishop, and to receive his left hand: people are constantly warned to be careful to avoid this when their children are about to be confirmed. ***Somerset UK*** [19]

~ A pregnant woman who stands godmother shouldn't lift Baby out of the font; else one of the children will die. ***Germany*** [1]

~ Children that cry at their christenings don't grow old. ***Germany*** [1]

~ The child crying at his christening is lucky, as the cries are evil spirits leaving his body. In St. Martin's Church, Canterbury, babies were brought into the church by the south entrance, and after the ceremony the north door was thrown open to permit the exit of evil spirits expelled by baptism. For in early times demons were believed to come from the north, where the Norse (Pagan) gods lived. ***UK*** [3]

~ A child sleeping at his baptism shows he'll not live long. ***Estonia*** [1]

~ Hair was cut off during christening, rolled up in wax and thrown in the font. The hair told fortunes: if the nubble stayed up, Baby would have a long life, if it didn't stay up, then Baby wouldn't be long for this world. ***Russia***

~ During baptism, they fix their eyes on Baby, to see if he holds his head up or lets it sink down. If up, he'll have a long life; if down, a short. ***Estonia*** [1]

~ If the church bells ring during the baptism of a baby less than one week of age, the child will become deaf. The only way to stop him from becoming deaf is to find a way of getting revenge on the bell ringer. ***France***

~ The godparents must not take hold of the chrism cloth by the corners. ***Germany***

~ Let Baby drink several teaspoonfuls of his own baptismal water as it will make him bright, and perhaps a good singer. ***German Pennsylvania USA***

~ Get a mite of bread consecrated so Baby's parents will never want for bread. ***Germany*** [1]

~ During the service, the father runs rapidly around the church, so the child may be gifted with fleetness of foot. ***Estonia*** [1]

~ Let the father put a sword in his baby's hand directly when he is christened, and Baby will be bold and brave. ***Germany*** [1]

~ The priest places a little salt in the child's mouth at baptism to impart wisdom. Hence the popular saying in regard to a person who is dull of understanding, that the priest put 'but little salt in his mouth.' ***Sicily*** [3]

~ A plate of salt was taken into the church for additional protection against evil. The use of salt at baptism in the Christian Church dates from the fourth century. It was an early practice to place blessed salt in Baby's mouth, to symbolise the counteraction of the sinfulness of Baby's nature. In the baptismal ceremonies of the Church in mediaeval times, salt, over which an exorcism had been said, was placed in the child's mouth, and his ears and nostrils were touched with saliva; practices which became obsolete about the time of the reign of Henry VIII. An octagonal font of the fifteenth century, in St. Margaret's Church, Ipswich, Suffolk, has upon one of its sides the figure of an angel bearing a scroll, on which appears a partially illegible inscription containing the words 'Sal et Saliva.' ***UK*** [3]

~ If by bribing the sexton they can get the baptismal water, they dash it as high as they can up the wall. The child will then attain high honours. ***Estonia*** [1]

~ Remove freckles by washing them with baptismal water. ***German Pennsylvania: USA***

~ If a girl anoints her lips with some stolen baptism oil and puts it into her lamps, the man who kisses her,

'Will be seized with a wild, strange love;
He'll heed not the dark world beneath him,
He'll heed not the heaven above.' ***Italy*** [46]

~ On arriving home from Church, a father holds his newly baptised child over the threshold for a while, to place Baby under the protection of the domestic divinities. ***Lithuania*** [3]

~ An egg and a prayer book were placed in the threshold, so the child crossing it after his baptism becomes as firm as the egg and a good Christian. ***Russian & Greek Orthodox***

~ For a child to grow up good, his godmother or the woman carrying home from church must immediately lay him under the table. Then Dad must pick him up and hand him to Mum. ***Germany*** [1]

~ Harm will come to the child if Friday churned butter, or Friday laid eggs are put into his christening cake. ***UK***

~ For three days following the baptism, Baby should not be bathed. The water from the first bath after the baptism should be used to water flowers. ***Greek Orthodox***

~ Three days after birth, the godfather shall 'buy' the child's crying from it by dropping a coin in Baby's swathings. ***Germany*** [1]

~ A man and a woman that have the same godparent shouldn't marry, because in the eyes of the Church they are brother and sister. ***Greek Orthodox***

PART V
BABYCARE

CHAPTER 20
NAMING BABY

~ In ancient times, naming a child meant bestowing a blessing or curse, as Baby's name was thought to prophesy his character. ***Jewish***

~ A name can influence everything that happens in a person's life. ***China***

~ Naming a child after a late relative makes the child doomed to an early death, as he'll be called away by the spirit of the dead (*UK*), brings bad luck to the child (*USA*), or means the deceased will be there in spirit looking after Baby. (*Europe & USA*)

~ It's bad luck to name Baby after a living relative. ***Ashkenazi Jews & I Kung Tribe Namibia***

~ When you name a baby after someone in the family, you need to get permission from the person 'owning' that name. If no permission is given, the child will have a life of misfortune. ***Hawaii***

~ The parents' names are never given, for that's unlucky. ***Japan***

~ If the first children take their parents' names, they will die before their parents. ***Germany*** [1]

~ It's unlucky to call a child by name before he is christened. ***UK***

~ Baby isn't given a name until he is old enough to talk. ***Washo Tribe: USA***

~ A fortune-teller picks a name for the baby. He selects a name that somehow makes up for any deficiencies the child might have in his spiritual make-up. E.g. if the child seems timid, a name is chosen to invoke courage. ***China***

~ Catholics tend to name their babies after one of their numerous Saints. The saint is said to especially look after child. A priest can refuse to give a 'Christian baptism' to a child, if no Saint of the desired name exists. ***Roman Catholic***

~ When a pregnant woman was near her due date, a deceased ancestor appeared to her in a dream to inform her which dead person was to be born again in her infant, and whose name Baby was therefore to take. If the woman had no such dream, Dad or the relatives determined the name by divination. ***Lapland*** [14]

~ A priest of Ifa, the god of divination, determines which ancestral soul has been reborn in Baby. As soon as this is decided, the parents are told the child must conform in all respects to the manner of life of the ancestor who now animates him, and if, as often happens, they profess ignorance, the priest supplies the necessary information. The child usually receives the name of this ancestor.' ***The Yorubas: Nigeria*** [14]

~ On the seventh day, a priest drops grains of rice into a cup of water, naming with each grain a deceased ancestor. From the movements of the seed in the water, and from observing Baby, the priest declares which ancestor has reappeared in the baby. The child generally receives the name of that ancestor. ***The Khonds India*** [14]

~ Eight days after the child is born, the shaman gives a naming ceremony where Baby is assigned a name and protective spirit. Newborns are given the names of recently deceased ancestors, and the qualities of the dead person are believed to be taken on by Baby. If the baby is unwanted, he may be killed within the eight days; traditionally it wasn't considered murder as Baby was still nameless. ***Inuit Eskimo***

~ Seven bananas are dubbed with names and laid before the infant. Baby is given the name allotted to the banana he grabs first. ***Kelantan Malaysia*** [22]

~ Baby's name is chosen by reading a Chinese calendar (Toong San) and Bai San (prayer) to ask if the name chosen is okay. If the name is too strong for the child, he'll get sick all the time and doctors won't be able to treat his illness. ***China***

~ Names are carefully chosen according to numerology and astrology. For boys, names with an even number of syllables are best. If you want a holy child, his name should contain four syllables. The name of a girl should contain three syllables. The name should be easy to pronounce, pleasing to hear, of clear meaning, and charming, ending in a long vowel. The syllables of the name are based on numerology. Names of gods and goddesses are preferred as the parents will then have the added blessing of remembering the deity each time they mention their child's name. ***Hindi***

~ On his 20th day, Baby is taken to the Mesa cliff and held up facing the rising sun. When the sun hits the baby, he is given his name. (*Hopi Tribe USA*) The tribe hold the child to the sun during his naming ceremony so the radiance of the sun will follow the child throughout life. (*Blackfoot Tribe USA*)

~ A baby doesn't thrive if you call him 'mite' or 'jackal'. If you call children 'little old man' or 'little old woman' they'll be stunted, and have premature wrinkles on their foreheads. Don't call a young child 'little crab' either, for he'll be stunted, as crabs crawl backwards. ***Germany*** [1]

~ If Baby has thirteen letters in his name, he'll have the devil's luck. Jack the Ripper, Charles Manson, Jeffrey Dahmer, Theodore Bundy and Albert De Salvo all had thirteen letters in their names. ***USA***

~ The spirit of the father's clan enters the baby early in pregnancy. However, the spirit of the mother's clan doesn't enter Baby until the naming ceremony, which takes place several months after the child is born. ***Africa***

~ The baby is baptised in the hospital's chapel soon after birth. All baby girls are baptised 'Maria' after the virgin mother. The name Maria is on all girls' baptismal certificates, but not on any legal documents. ***Spain***

~ The child is given two names, one based on the constellation at the time of birth, and the other for day-to-day use. ***Bangladesh***

~ A month or two after Baby is born, a naming ceremony is held around the full or new moon. Some children are given two names, one to use in their normal lives, and a special name used only within their circle. ***Pagan***

NAME NUMEROLOGY

Letters of the alphabet are said to have a vibratory frequency that can be matched with the vibratory frequency of numbers. Therefore, each letter of the alphabet is given a numerical value. Before giving Baby a name, many people will check the name's numerological value to see if it's fitting. If the 'birth date' or 'life path' number (see page 112) has revealed any inherent character weakness, a name can be chosen for Baby with a numerological value to try to compensate for this weakness.

THE DESTINY NUMBER

This number describes Baby's potential, the talents and attitudes at his disposal in his lifetime. The Destiny number is what Baby *should* do. The number is derived from all the letters in the FULL BIRTH NAME as it appears on the birth certificate. To arrive at the Destiny number, take each name separately and add up the letter values using the conversion chart below. Reduce each name to a single digit or to a master number which is not reduced further (11 or 22). Then add the results of all of the names to arrive at a total which you then once again reduce to a single digit or master number.

1	2	3	4	5	6	7	8	9
A	B	C	D	E	F	G	H	I
J	K	L	M	N	O	P	Q	R
S	T	U	V	W	X	Y	Z	

Example of Expression Number: SHAUN THOMAS FRANKLIN

SHAUN = 1+8+1+3+5=18 =9

THOMAS = 2+8+6+4+1+1=22 (a master number that is not reduced further)

FRANKLIN = 6+9+1+5+2+3+9+5=40=4

The Expression number is 9+22+4=35 and 35 reduces to 8. Shaun's expression Number is therefore 8.

THE SOUL URGE NUMBER

The Soul Urge Number denotes what Baby will *value* most regardless of his Life Path Number (what he *is* from birth calculated from birth date) or his Destiny Number (what he *should* become in life). It's calculated from all of the vowels in the full birth name as recorded on the birth certificate, converted to numbers, and reduced to a single number or a master number. Here's a chart reflecting the number value of the vowels and 'sometime' vowels:

1	2	3	4	5	6	7	8	9
A	-	-	-	E	-	-	-	I
-	-	-	-	-	O	-	-	-
-	-	U	-	W*	-	Y*	-	-

* A **Y** is also a vowel when there is no other vowel in a syllable (Lynn or Carolyn) and when it's preceded by a vowel and sounded as one sound (Hayden). A **W** is treated as a vowels when it's preceded by a vowel and produces a single sound, as in such names and Bradshaw.[61]

Much has been written on numerology elsewhere so I will not go into detail regarding the meaning of the numbers here. The numbers meanings can easily be obtained in books and on websites such as www.astrology-numerology.com

Chapter 21
Babycare

~ The baby is 'smoked' in fragrant smoke in a special ceremony to make him healthy and strong. Bark of the Gubanu tree is burnt and then made into a special charcoal paste that is rubbed onto his skin. ***Aborigine***
~ Don't step over Baby when he's on the floor or he'll be stepped on all his life. ***China***
~ Don't hold Baby with your bare hands or pick him up all the time, or he'll become very spoiled. ***Thailand***
~ Baby must be carried quite flat for his first twelve weeks. Baby should be carried in the arms twice a day for thirty minutes. ***Edwardian UK*** [27]
~ Everyone passes Baby around so he'll be generous, and always surrounded by happiness, friends and family. ***Navajo Tribe***
~ 'A baby's brain needs to be kept from all unnecessary impressions, sudden noises, etc, and he should be but little talked to. This may sound harsh, but is a necessary warning to young mothers…An excited baby leads to many serious nervous diseases, and a good plan for the first three months is to keep Baby away from his brothers and sisters who wish to play with him.' ***Edwardian UK***[27]
~ Loud noises are discouraged around Baby. A loud noise such as the slamming of a door could cause the soft spot on his head to collapse. If this happens, take Baby, turn him upside down by grabbing his legs and pound the bottom of his feet. This will pop the soft spot back out. ***Spain***
~ Weighing Baby is unlucky. Doing so is an insult to God, from whom the child has come; God may take the child back as a punishment. ***Slavic***
~ To weigh Baby before he's a year old is testing fate; Baby could die prematurely or grow up stunted. ***UK***
~ Never say Baby is heavy as only dead people are heavy. ***Trinidad & Tobago***
~ It's not good to hit an animal with the same whip that has been used to discipline a child. ***Germany*** [1]
~ Beating a daughter on her buttocks causes her to become sexually hyperactive and causes many domestic problems. Avoid mistreating one's daughter or she'll be mistreated later on by her husband. ***Indonesia***
~ According to their saying, 'a hurt baby is more lovable' and mothers who feel affectionate toward their babies often slap, squeeze, or bite them until the babies burst into tears. ***Inuit: Eskimo*** [62]
~ It's forbidden to hang a picture or keep a picture of any being that possesses a soul. The Prophet prohibited having pictures in houses and declared all the picture makers would go to hell. For every picture made, a soul is created and

punished. ***Islamic***
~ Bastard children are luckier than lawful ones. If your first godchild is illegitimate, you'll be lucky in marriage. ***Germany*** [1]
~ Baby's mouth should be closed for him, and the good habit of breathing through the nose established early on. Tonsils can become enlarged, and the throat become rough and dry if this advice isn't heeded. ***Edwardian UK*** [27]
~ A babysitter should never clean their teeth while 'sitting'. ***India***
~ Rub apple on Baby's tongue so he can sing well. ***Southern USA***
~ Don't let Baby tread barefoot on a table as he'll get sore feet. ***Germany*** [1]
~ If you sweep a circle around a baby, he or she will never marry. ***Italy***
~ If an older child gets jealous of the baby, Mum should let him take a shower between her legs. ***Thailand***
~ A child must not be passed through a window, or Mum will have another child before the end of a year.
~ If a baby stands too soon, it will cause him to be bowlegged. ***UK & USA***
~ As soon as Baby turns onto his stomach for the first time, put a bowl of water on his back. ***Thailand***
~ The first laugh is an important event, and the person who makes a baby laugh for the first time must host a dinner on his behalf. At the dinner, the mother holds a wedding basket containing earth salt. When people pass by with their plates full of food, the mother places a piece of earth salt in her baby's right hand and helps him put it on the food. This introduces him to a lifelong sense of obligation to the family, clan, and people. ***Navajo Tribe USA***
~ Don't allow Baby to sit up much for nine months lest his spine bend in the wrong direction; let him lie flat and kick, propped up slightly with pillows if he's bored. ***Edwardian UK*** [27]
~ If you make a promise to a child and don't uphold it, he'll have a bad fall. ***Germany*** [1]
~ If Baby falls over, hit the floor repeatedly to comfort him and say it will make him grow faster. ***Thailand***
~ If the temperature is less than 60 degrees Fahrenheit, Baby must not be let out the house until at least six months old. If it's winter, you will just have to wait until spring before the child can go out. At six months old, Baby should be wrapped up in his pram and taken out in the fresh air. A winter schedule is between 11am until 1pm and 2pm until 3.30pm. This strengthens his constitution. ***Edwardian UK*** [27]
~ Baby shouldn't be allowed to crawl as this is what beasts and savages do. ***17th Century UK***
~ If a child under a year old is taken into the cellar, he'll grow up timid. ***Germany*** [1]
~ Baby's spirit nature may occasionally wander off on its own. When Mum

carries her very young infant along a pathway and meets a cross-path, she'll break off a leaf from an adjoining bush, and throw it on the cross-path so Baby's Spirit must follow her and not go off in another direction. ***Moruca River Indians Guyana*** [21]

~ If Baby points a finger at the moon, he'll get a wooden finger (***Germany*** [1]) or he'll lose his ears. (***Taiwan***)

~ Children must not stretch their forefinger towards heaven; they kill a dear little angel every time. ***Germany*** [1]

~ Never let a child point at a grave. ***Madagascar***

~ Baby's spirit nature doesn't usually free itself from Mum until he begins to crawl or walk. Therefore, up until this time, whatever affects Mum in the way of food or otherwise, exerts a corresponding influence on Baby. ***Moruca River Indians*** [21]

~ Baby has a celebration after one lunar year called 'quitting the cradle.' This is a party attended by numerous guests. Baby sits on a bed surrounded by various objects such as scissors, flowers, books, and pencils. The item he picks up first determines his future vocation. If he takes the scissors, hell become a tailor; the book, a learned man, and so on. ***Vietnam***

~ To learn about Baby's future, place a book, a few coins and a bottle in front of him. If he reaches for the book, he'll be a scholar, if he reaches for the coins, he'll be wealthy, if he reaches for the bottle, he'll be a drunk. ***Germany***

~ On his first birthday, one kilogram of rice cake is tied onto Baby's back. The child carries it around as a sign of health and strength. ***Japan***

~ Potty training should begin at one year's old. Place Baby on a potty for ten minutes at a fixed time twice a day. ***Edwardian UK*** [27]

SWADDLING

~ Babies must be tightly tied up so they don't not grow 'crooked' or 'evil shaped'. Their heads must be firmly tied down, or they might throw off their heads from their shoulders [63] and if not swaddled tightly, Baby will tear his ears off, scratch his eyes out, break his legs, play with his genitals, become overly aggressive, or fall to pieces. ***UK***

~ Baby was wrapped in a blanket and tied into a bamboo basket until he was three or four years old. ***Japan***

~ Each tribe had their own cradleboard (baby carrier). Baby was kept swaddled tightly in it for most of the time. The curved headboard was known as the rainbow, and when a child was laced into the cradleboard, he was said to be 'under the rainbow.' The flat boards were believed to give Baby a strong, straight back, and the soft supporting pads helped Baby form a nicely rounded head. The cradleboard was blessed with corn pollen, prayers, songs and good thoughts for Baby. ***Navajo Tribe USA***

Babycare

CRYING

~ When Baby cries at night, his mother should sing or talk louder than Baby's voice to avoid spirits taking away Baby's voice. *Guyana*
~ A baby that doesn't cry when born will hold back his feelings. Whereas a newborn that is vocal will be strongly opinionated. *UK*
~ If Baby cries a lot in his first three months, wrap his stomach tightly so no air can get in. *Thailand*
~ Let Baby cry as it strengthens his lungs. Babies who cry loud and long live long.
~ A child that cries a lot could be a changeling.
~ The 'Holy Godmother' teaches Baby to smile, and crying means Baby is being punished for stubbornness. *Vietnam*
~ A child crying on his first birthday will always be unhappy.

TO STOP BABY CRYING

~ Place Baby on your lap, grab his hands and pull them down towards his feet. *Italy*
~ Hold Baby's leg with one hand, and hit the wall with the other. *Faroe Isles*
~ Hold Baby in the air by the hands and feet and then let go of his feet. *Italy*
~ Take Baby's shirt off and wave it over the fire. Then put his shirt back on. *Hmong*
~ Get a piece of clothing from the oldest sibling, face Baby north, and swing the clothing around him three times counter-clockwise. *Poland*
~ Put three keys in Baby's cradle *Germany* [1]
~ Catnip tea, tea made of the white of chicken's droppings, and cloths dipped in sugar water quiet Baby. *USA*
~ If Baby cries much in the first six weeks, pull him three times through a piece of unboiled yarn in silence. If that does no good, let Mum, after being churched, go home in silence, undress in silence, and throw all her clothes on the cradle backwards. *Germany* [1]
~ A baby cries a lot because someone has cast the 'evil eye' on him. To counter this curse, the family must find the perpetrator, and then wrap Baby in that person's sweaty shirt. Only then will Baby calm down. *Hondorus*
~ Babies who continuously cry are disturbed by evil spirits and to ward these off, a single Pomelo leaf should be placed beneath the cot mattress. *China*
~ If Baby is cross, he must be possessed. Take him before sunrise to a pond and dip him in three times to cleanse him of evil spirits. *Newfoundland*
~ A fretful baby longs for something for which Mum had an ungratified craving for during pregnancy. The only remedy is to find out what this is, and give Baby a taste of it. *Pennsylvania USA*
~ If Baby cries continually, he should be smoked over a fire made of the nest of a weaverbird, bottle gourd skin, and a piece of wood that has been struck by

lightning. ***Malaysia*** [22]

~ If you believe the wailing infant is a changeling say, 'Stop that music, lad, or I'll put thee on the fire.' If he starts again, 'Art thou at it again, piper of the one tune? Let me hear that music any more from thee, and I will kill thee with the dirk (dagger).' The fairy will take such a fright that he'll keep quiet a good while. ***Scotland*** [59]

~ When Baby is subject to convulsive weeping or spasms, and loses sleep, Mum takes a straw from his sleeping place and puts it into her mouth. Then, while she is fumigated with dried cow dung, into which her husband's and her hair has been mingled, she chants:

'Hair, hair, burn!
Dirt and hair burn
Dirt and hair burn
Illness be burned!' ***Romany Gypsy*** [7]

~ Convulsive weeping in children is cured as follows: In the evening, Mum carries Baby three times around the fire on which is burning a pippin full of water with three coals. With this water, she washes Baby's head, and pours some of it on a black dog. Then she goes to the stream, and drops a red twist into it, saying:

'Nivashi take this twist, and with it the weeping of my child. When it's well I will bring thee apples and eggs'. ***Hungarian Gypsy*** [7]

BABY'S SLEEP

~ Never sweep a room where a baby sleeps or the 'dream soul', which leaves the body during sleep, will be swept away also. ***Africa***

~ It's unlucky and possibly fatal to the child's health to watch a baby sleeping. ***Jewish***

~ It's good luck to see a baby smiling in his sleep. ***Newfoundland***

~ A smile on a sleeping child may be a sign the angels are playing with him. ***German Pennsylvania***

~ Until the child is one year old, he speaks with God and the angels. The Angels show Baby golden fruit in his sleep; if Baby can grasp the fruit, Baby laughs; if he can't, he weeps. ***Romanian Jews***

~ When a child laughs in his sleep, he's playing with the Angel of Death or Lilith; therefore, he should be lightly tapped on the mouth. ***Jewish***

~ When children laugh in their sleep, or open and turn their eyes, 'the Jüdel plays with them'. If the Jüdel won't let Baby sleep, give the Jüdel something to play with. Buy a new little pot, pour Baby's bathwater in it, and set it on the oven: in a few days, the Jüdel will have sucked every drop out. Sometimes eggshells, out of which the yolk has been blown into the child's pap and the mother's caudle, are hung on the cradle by a thread, for the Jüdel to play with instead of the child. ***Germany*** [1]

Babycare

~ If Baby sleeps on through a thunderstorm, the lightning will not strike. ***Germany*** [1]

~ Anyone who carries a basket into the room of a woman recovering from childbirth must break a splinter from it and place it in the cradle; otherwise he'll take Mum's or Baby's sleep away. ***Germany & Jewish***

~ So Baby may not be robbed of sleep and rest, a stranger shall sit down when he comes into the room and nobody should remove utensils of any kind from the house, especially those holding burning coals. ***Germany*** [1]

~ When going to bed, leave nothing lying on the table, else the oldest or youngest in the house can get no sleep. ***Germany*** [1]

~ The mother placed an open Holy Bible under the pillow of a sleepless child,
'*and there is treasure kept,
While one short, fervent, prayer she said,
And lol her darling sweetly, slept!*' ***German Pennsylvania***

~ If a child suffers from sleeplessness, some of his mother's hair should be sewed into his wrappings, and others pulverized, mixed with an elderberry decoction, and given him to drink. ***Romany Gypsy*** [7]

~ When children are bewitched and can't sleep, take some earth off the common and throw it over them. Or put under Baby's pillow straw that breeding women lay under their backs; only you must get it away from them without saying a word. ***Germany*** [1]

~ If Baby can't sleep, it's because of evil spirits. A healer rolls a chicken egg (a symbol of the life-force) over Baby to cleanse his soul. The egg is cracked open into a glass of water. If the egg-white is cloudy, that's the evil taken from Baby's body. ***Mexico***

~ Cuba is the Goddess of infant's sleep and Cunina is the Goddess of infants in the cradle. ***Ancient Rome***

BABY'S BED

~ During the second trimester of pregnancy, Vogul women build a trough-like cradle out of birch bark. The newborn sleeps in it for one week under a covering of swanskin or under a covering of hare fur in winter. Once ceremonially purified, Baby moves to a permanent cradle and the first cradle is hung in the woods with all the other first cradles belonging to the town's children. ***Siberia***

~ In rural areas, the cradle is made from Peachtree wood to give Baby long life. ***China***

~ The first cradle must be fully paid for before being brought into the house, lest it cause the child to die a pauper and be too poor to pay for his own coffin. ***UK***

~ A fetish in the form of a cradle made of nine kinds of wood brings luck to the child who sleeps in it. ***Bosnian Gypsy*** [7]

~ Don't place the foot of Baby's bed facing the door, as it means death. **USA**
~ Babies sleep best with their heads to the north and their feet to the south. Turn the cot around north to south if Baby is sick. ***Jewish, USA, Europe***
~ A newborn shouldn't be laid on his left side first or he'll be clumsy. ***Germany*** [1]
~ Never rock an empty cradle: it rocks Baby's rest away (*Germany*[1]), it's unlucky (*Jewish, Slavic, UK & USA*), it foretells the death of a child (*Caithness Scotland*) or causes Baby to get colic or pleurisy. (*German Pennsylvania*)
~ If two people rock one child, he is robbed of his rest. ***Germany*** [1]
~ Never change Baby's bed on Friday, or turn his mattress on a Sunday, as he'll have bad dreams. **UK**
~ It brings good luck to sleep on unironed sheets.
~ When making the bed, don't interrupt your work or a restless night will be spent in it.
~ Air Baby's bedding for an hour each day, first in front of the window, then in front of the fire. ***Edwardian UK*** [27]
~ Good housewives make the beds in the morning; lazy ones at noon; slatterns and pigs at night. ***German Pennsylvania***
~ Put a bible under Baby's pillow and his bad dreams will go away. **USA**
~ Never hand things over a cradle with the child in it; nor leave it open. To stretch over the cradle causes tension of the heart. ***Germany***
~ If Mum doesn't want any more children, she should keep the cradle, or some of her last baby's clothes. **UK**

YAWNING
~ When Baby yawns, the devil is laughing at him. ***Islamic*** [20]
~ Make the sign of the cross over his mouth or an evil spirit will rush down his mouth and take up abode there. ***Greece & Ireland***
~ Place the hand, palm outwards, before the mouth to stop any demons entering. ***Turkestan*** [3]

SNEEZING
~ A baby sneezing is greeted with fervent benedictions, such as, 'The blessing of God and the holy Mary be upon you!' to counteract the scheming of evil disposed fairies. ***Ireland***
~ Anyone sneezing places himself in the power of a witch, unless another invokes a divine blessing. ***Holland*** [3]
~ The Devil can enter Baby's body when he sneezes. Having someone say, 'God bless you' drives Satan away. ***Europe***
~ Grandmothers must exclaim, 'God help you!' when they hear their grandchild sneeze. ***Midlands UK*** [5]
~ Sneezing is a bad omen because it indicates the indwelling spirit is about to

quit the body, affording an opportunity for a homeless spirit to enter and cause illness. (*Ewe Tribes Africa*[31]*)* A similar belief leads the Calabar natives to exclaim, 'Far from you!' when anyone sneezes, with an appropriate gesture as if throwing off evil. (*Africa*)

~ Sneezing is an ominous sign and should be accompanied by a pious ejaculation, asking God's forgiveness. ***Islamic***

~ A newborn is considered by his nurse to be in the fairy spells until he has sneezed. 'God sain (save) the bairn,' exclaimed an old Scottish nurse when her little charge sneezed at length, 'it's no a warlock.' ***Scotland*** [3]

~ To cure a fairy-stricken child, certain herbs are thrown on a fire. After a thick smoke has risen, Baby is carried thrice around the fire while an incantation is repeated and holy water is sprinkled liberally about. Meantime all doors must be closed, lest some inquisitive fairy spy upon the proceedings; and the magical rites must be continued until the child sneezes three times, for this looses the spell, permanently redeeming Baby from the witch's power. ***Ireland*** [15]

~ Islanders believe that when the spirit goes travelling about, its return naturally occasions some commotion, as is evident from the violent act of sneezing. They therefore deem it proper to welcome back the wandering spirit, the form of greeting varying in the different islands. The phrase employed by Raratonga natives is 'Ha! You have come back!' ***South Pacific*** [3]

~ Sneezing 'into the air' allows the soul to escape and death could be imminent, therefore always cover the nose with your hand.

~ When someone sneezes, his soul temporally leaves his body. ***Malaysia***

~ Those who sneezed were congratulated, as it was believed a violent sneeze expelled evil. ***UK***

~ Somebody must be speaking evil of the one who sneezed, or he's being talked about ***Mexico*** [3]

~ One sneeze indicates that someone is praising Baby, while two sneezes mean the opposite. ***Japan*** [3]

~ When Baby sneezes, someone is calling his name, either with good or evil intent, the motive being shown by the character of the sneeze. A gentle sneeze implies kindly intent, while a violent sneeze indicates bad intent. ***The Banks Islands Polynesia*** [3]

~ The Supreme Judge of the spiritual world is continually turning over the pages of a book containing accounts of the life and deeds of every human being; and when he comes to the page relating to any individual, the latter never fails to sneeze. The accompanying expression is, 'May the judgment be favourable to you.' ***Siam & Laos*** [3]

~ 'If you sneeze on a Monday, you sneeze for danger;
Sneeze on a Tuesday, kiss a stranger;

Sneeze on a Wednesday, sneeze for a letter;
Sneeze on a Thursday, something better;
Sneeze on a Friday, sneeze for sorrow;
Sneeze on a Saturday, see your sweetheart tomorrow.
Sneeze on a Sunday, and the devil will have domination over you all week.'
~ *'One for sorrow*
Two for joy
Three for a letter
Four for a boy.
Five for silver
Six for gold
Seven for a secret, never to be told'
~ A young child's sneeze has a certain mystic significance, and is intimately associated with his prospective welfare or ill luck. When Baby sneezes, Mum immediately recites a long charm of words. If the sneeze occurs during a meal, it predicts the arrival of a visitor, or some interesting news. ***Maori*** [3]
~ If Baby's sneeze occurs during a meal, it's an evil omen. ***Tonga*** [3]
~ If they sneeze in first getting out of bed in the morning, visitors will be there in the course of the day, in numbers corresponding to the times they sneeze. ***Selkirkshire Scotland***
~ Even educated people maintain that idiots are incapable of sneezing, and hence, the inference is clear; sneezing is evidence of the possession of a certain degree of intelligence. ***Scotland*** [3]
~ Three sneezes are unlucky. ***Turkestan*** [3]
~ When someone sneezes, he's blessed as it is proof the ancestral spirit is within him. ***Zulu Tribe Africa*** [3]

KISSING

~ Children who haven't yet learned to speak are forbidden from kissing each other lest it makes them mute (*Russia*) or causes one of them to die. (*Germany*[1])
~ Kissing Baby on the lips makes him speak sooner (*Turkey*), or causes him to have a hard time in cutting his teeth. (*USA, Holland & Germany*)
~ If you kiss a sleeping baby, you make him conceited (*Zanzibar*) or curse him into being an overly sensitive adult who is easily offended. (*Philippines*)
~ When a baby is kissed on the soles of his feet, he'll walk early. ***Turkey***
~ A child should not be kissed on the feet, since this is the custom of asking the dead for forgiveness. ***Jewish***
~ A child that's kissed too much when young may suffer through a lack of the same in his older years. ***German Pennsylvania***
~ Babies kissed on the back of the neck will become obstinate. ***Turkey***
~ Never kiss a child on his hands, as he'll grow up supersensitive. ***Philippines***

~ Don't kiss a newborn when leaving the house, or you'll take his dream away. ***Hungary***
~ If an unmarried woman kisses a baby on the ninth day after his birth, the next man she kisses will be her husband. ***Italy***

GROWTH

~ Crawling through windows stunts Baby's growth. (There's a rule that having crawled out through the window, Baby must crawl back in again to break the spell.) (*Creole USA & German Pennsylvania*)
~ A child under three, pushed in through a peep window, stops growing. ***Germany*** [1]
~ When a child is taken out of doors, don't keep the upper half of the door closed, or he'll stop growing. ***Germany*** [1]
~ Permitting a child to crawl, or walk between a man's legs stops his growth. ***German Pennsylvania***
~ Never jump over a child, or he'll remain short. ***Turkey***
~ Stepping over a child stops his growth, therefore, whoever takes such a step must step back again to break the spell. ***Jewish & German Pennsylvania***
~ If you walk over a child's feet while he's sitting or lying down, you will stunt his growth. ***Belize***
~ Never pass anything over Baby's head as he won't grow; to break the spell, pull the hair on top of his head upwards. ***Estonia***[1]
~ Two babies can't be left alone in a room together without completing their fortieth day; otherwise, one will become tall and the other will become short. ***Turkey***
~ An Ojebway is afraid that if he repeats his own name it will prevent his growth, and he'll be consequently small in stature. ***Ojebway Indians USA*** [14]
~ Payment of the doctor's fee in full prevents a child from growing. ***German Pennsylvania USA***
~ Frequent stretching out on the bare floor aids young children to attain greater length.
~ If you shine a light into the face of a sleeping child, he'll grow taller.
~ If children are dwarfish, their nail clippings cut on a Friday should be burnt, and the ashes put into their food to make them grow. ***Romany Gypsy*** [7]
~ Wild ginger is given to a child to make him grow fast. ***Hupa Indians California*** [29]

TEETHING

~ The first tooth signifies a child is thriving; a safe time to anticipate his first steps. Whoever discovers Baby's first tooth must buy his first shoes. ***Ireland***
~ Baby's mental development is linked to how early teething starts. ***USA & UK***

~ If Baby's first tooth appears on his lower jaw, he'll have a long life.
~ Teething causes diarrhoea, wheezing, nappy rash and high fever. **USA & UK**
~ The more difficult the teething period is for Baby, the better he'll be for it.
~ The longer Baby has to wait for his teeth, the longer he'll have them in his old age. **West Country UK**
~ Don't say 'the first tooth comes up' rather say 'the flower comes up'. **Thailand**
~ A baby's tooth, set in a ring or brooch, should be worn to bring good luck.
~ When the first tooth is cut, Mum must tap it with a silver spoon, to make Baby rich. **Bulgaria**
~ When Baby is six months old, Mum makes a special ritual 'banya' (sauna) to celebrate the age when Baby usually gets his first tooth, and therefore his own soul. **Karelia Russia**

CHARMS TO AID TEETHING

~ Give Baby an egg the first time he comes into a house to help him teeth. **Germany** [1]
~ For easy teething, Mum should, for three Sundays, leave church silently and blow into Baby's mouth. **France**[1]
~ If Baby rides on a black foal, he'll cut his teeth quickly. **Germany** [1]
~ Putting on Baby's left sock first, and putting on his right coat sleeve first, helps his teething. **German Pennsylvania USA**
~ If a woman getting up from her childbed lace a crust of bread on her, and make her child a zuller or schlotzer of it, Baby won't have toothache. **Germany** [1]
~ When you see a child's first tooth, immediately box his ear, and he'll cut the rest of his teeth easier. **Germany** [1]
~ A mouse's head bitten off with teeth or cut off with gold and hung on a child's neck, helps him teethe. **Germany** [1]
~ Painful teething is relieved by wearing a cowrie shell amulet (*UK*), a fossil shark's tooth (*Celtic*), a dime on a piece of string around Baby's neck (*African American*) a bear's tooth and silver whistle (*Germany* [7]) or a coral necklace (*Cornwall*)
~ Rub Baby's gums with dog's milk (*Medieval UK*), whiskey or brandy (*African American*), boiled rabbit's brain (*German Pennsylvania*), cinnamon (*Creole USA*), cyperas with butter and oil-of-lilies (*Medieval UK,*) a paste made with cloves and vanilla (*African American*), honey, salt and oil (*Medieval UK*) or a mixture of chicken fat and hare's brain.
~ Rub the tooth or gum with a snakeskin (*German Pennsylvania*), or Mum's gold wedding ring to ease discomfort. (*Yorkshire UK*)
~ Cure toothache with a piece of white bread marked with a cross laid against the gum. **16th Century UK**

Babycare

~ Blow tobacco smoke in Baby's mouth to ease teething pain. ***African American***
~ 'Bathe Baby's head a while, with water boiled with camomile.' ***Medieval UK***
~ Charm for teeth:
'Christ pass'd by his brother's door
Saw his brother lying on the floor
What aileth thee brother?
Pain in thy teeth?
Thy teeth shall pain thee no more,
In the name of the Father, Son and Holy Ghost.' ***Cornwall UK*** [12]

TALKING

~ Never tickle Baby's feet or you'll make him stutter. ***UK, USA, Holland & Germany***
~ Don't buy your children rattles, nor allow any to be given, or they'll be slow in learning to talk. ***Germany*** [1]
~ For tongue-tied children it's good to eat beggar's bread. If a child is backward in speaking, take two loaves that have stuck together in baking, and break them loose over his head. ***Germany*** [1]
~ If the godfather's letter is opened over Baby's mouth, Baby will speak early. ***Germany*** [1]
~ If you give a child an egg the first time he comes into a house it makes him talkative. Rainwater also makes children talk early. ***Germany*** [1]
~ Children should be seen and not heard. ***Victorian UK***
~ The Roman God Locutius taught children to speak.
~ Patron Saint of Children Learning to Speak: Zeno of Verona
~ Patron Saint of Stammering Children: Notkar Balbulus

WALKING

~ When Baby makes his first step, relatives must cut the invisible cord which could hinder him. ***Bulgaria***
~ If a child won't learn to walk, make him creep silently on three Friday mornings through a raspberry bush grown into the ground at both ends. ***Germany*** [1]
~ To stimulate Baby to learn to walk quickly, Mum gets a tibi-tibi lizard and gets it to bite her baby's feet and knees; Baby is also incited to activity by putting a small stinging ant on him. ***Arawak Indians Guyana*** [21]
~ Wearing shoes will help a baby walk sooner. ***UK***
~ To make Baby walk early, rub the back of his legs with egg-white. ***Belize***
~ Should a child's legs seem inclined to bend, no walking should be allowed until a later date. ***Edwardian UK*** [27]

~ A child's first fall never hurts. **Germany** [1]
~ Embroider a cat's head on the shoes of a child just learning to walk to make him as surefooted as a cat. **China**
~ The pram should be used until Baby is four years old as over-walking brings on infant paralysis. **Edwardian UK** [27]
~ The author knows of a gentleman who did not walk until he was four. His parents believed that this would mean in older years he would be able to walk for longer. Now in his late seventies, he believes his continued agility is testament to this West Country belief. **Cornwall UK**
~ A baby is unable to walk until the soft spot on his head grows hard.
~ If a child has a date stone about him, he doesn't fall, or isn't hurt much. **Germany** [1]
~ Until Baby is able to walk well, Mum mustn't eat deer, turtle, or iguana; animals which for some days after birth, creep or crawl very slowly. If Mum eats their flesh, Baby will walk too slowly. **Pomeroon Arawaks: Guyana** [21]
~ The husband abstains from venison after his wife's delivery lest his baby walk too slowly. **The Akawai, Carib & Warrau Indians Guyana** [21]
~ The Roman God Statulinus helps babies to walk
~ Patron Saint of Children Learning to Walk: Zeno of Verona
~ Patron Saint of Children Late in Learning to Walk: Vaast

WEANING

~ At one month old, Baby has all his hair shaved off and is given chewed rice mixed with banana to eat. **Laos**
~ Baby's 100th day of life is considered lucky. The table is set with a four-course meal, and Baby is encouraged to touch the food with a spoon. **Japan**
~ Baby's first solid food is three spoonfuls of the custard-like flesh of a young coconut fed to him by a Buddhist priest. **Thailand**
~ Girls must be weaned by a waning moon to make them slim and delicate, or their breasts will be too large; boys at full moon, so they may grow big and strong; but no children during the passage of birds, else they'll be restless and changeable. **Lithuania**[1]
~ If a child is weaned during the waning of the moon, he'll decay all the time the moon continues to wane. **Angus Scotland** [64]
~ If Baby is weaned during the summer, he'll die young. **German Pennsylvania**
~ Mum should never wean Baby in the spring when trees are in blossom, especially when there is late snow on the ground as Baby is bound to get white hair prematurely. (*USA & Germany*) If weaned when the leaves fall, Baby will become bald very young. (*German Pennsylvania*)
~ Weaning should start on one of the church's holy days, ideally on Good Friday, or failing that, when the moon is on the wane. It shouldn't be

Babycare

attempted in the spring, or Baby will be prematurely grey-haired, and certainly not on Childermas Day. ***UK***

~ If a cow calves in the sign of Virgo, the calf will not live one year; if it happens in Scorpio, it will die much sooner; therefore to protect Baby from mortal inflammation, he must not be weaned during these signs. Neither should Baby be weaned in the sign of the Capricorn or Aquarius. ***Germany*** [24]

~ To wean a child, let the mother set him down on the floor, and knock him over with her foot; he'll forget her the sooner. ***Germany*** [1]

~ When Baby is weaning, give him three times a roll to eat, a penny to lose, and a key. ***Germany*** [1]

~ Educa is the Roman goddess of baby food and infants who are weaning.

~ Baby's first food is taken from a neighbour with the blessing, 'May this be the last time you are supported by others.' ***Eastern European Jews*** [2]

~ As the (unlucky) Last Supper was celebrated upstairs by Jesus and his disciples, all meals must take place on the ground floor for luck.

~ Don't blow on Baby's first pap so he won't scald his mouth on hot things in future. ***Germany*** [1]

~ Never stir Baby's food widdershins (against the sun). ***Celtic***

~ Eating from a silver spoon makes Baby healthier. ***Russia***

~ The left hand is never used for eating as the devil eats with the left hand. ***Islamic***

~ It's dangerous to let Baby eat any food that has been stepped over. ***Gypsy***

~ The first meat you should give a child is roast lark. ***Germany*** [1]

~ If you give Baby part of a red baked apple to eat the first time instead of pap, he'll have red cheeks. ***Germany*** [1]

~ You mustn't cut a banana, but simply break it with the fingers, because in cutting it you cut the cross. ***Creole USA***

~ It's not right for a child to eat kidney, or any part of one, before he can pronounce his own name distinctly. ***Isle of Man*** [44]

~ Don't give milk when Baby has a cold as it causes excessive phlegm. ***UK***

~ If a child spills milk on the ground, Mum shouldn't worry about it and say, 'That is to the fairies, leave it to them and welcome,' and the child must never be scolded lest it bring bad luck. This is where the saying 'Don't cry over spilled milk' comes from. ***Ireland***

~ Never let the child eat any fish from the head downward, as this is sure to turn heads of the fish away from the coasts and cause general bad luck. Rather let him eat it from tail to head. ***Cornish fishing communities*** [12]

~ Don't let Baby eat fish until he can say the word 'fish' to avoid him choking on fishbone. ***Thailand***

~ If the child can't or won't eat, give a little feast to the fowls of the air or a black dog. ***Germany*** [1]

Chapter 22
Grooming Baby

BATHING BABY

~ Care should be taken not to wash a newborn's right hand for the first three days as doing so washes his good luck away, particularly in financial matters. **UK**

~ Washing Baby's hands before his first birthday will make him poor all his life. It's also unlucky to wash Baby's head for the first twelve months. **Cornwall UK** [12]

~ Every newborn boy, before his first bath, is placed upon a horse, to impart manly qualities to him. The animal is specially brought into the room for this purpose. **Brandenburg Germany** [1]

~ A child's bathtub must not be used for any other purpose, or he'll not prosper. **Jewish**

~ The smaller the jug in which water is drawn for a baby girl's bath, the smaller her breasts will be. **Germany** [1]

~ Put three pennies in Baby's first bath, so he'll always have money; a pen, so he'll learn fast; a rosary, so he'll grow up pious; an egg, so he'll have a clear voice. But the three pennies and the egg must be given to the first beggar. **Germany** [1]

~ In Baby's first bath, put sugar and salt to make him a good, sweet, and well respected person (*Russia*), put salt to add taste to his speech and actions (*Yemen*), pieces of bread and sugar for luck (*Jewish & Slavic*), various tools and coins to make Baby a talented craftsman and rich (*Russia*), and a raw egg and gold bangles to bring strength and good fortune. (*Morocco*)

~ The first time Baby takes a bath, put a little water in his mouth so he'll always be calm around water. **Portugal**

~ Chuck out Baby's first bath water to get rid of any bad energy.

~ Empty the bathwater under a green tree, and the children will stay fresh. **Germany** [1]

~ Water from Baby' first bath should be deposited under a tree in leaf to promote the child's healthy growth.

~ If the first bath water is thrown over the roots of a tree in bloom, Baby will always be good-looking. **Wales**

~ A Newborn's bath water is emptied in the most remote spot, lest many trample on it and the child is downtrodden and despised. **Estonia & Iceland**

~ Baby's ears should not be washed for the first six weeks as it causes deafness. **Russia**

~ Washing Baby's face in his own urine makes him handsome. **German Pennsylvania**

Babycare

~ Potatoes will grow behind Baby's ears if that area isn't washed properly. ***UK***
~ Don't keep putting the bathing towel on and off the child, or he'll have no abiding place when old. ***Germany*** [1]
~ When Baby is one month old, his bath is sprinkled with the petals of seven different flowers for good luck. ***Indonesia***
~ Baby's head is to be daily washed in rum to harden his skull. ***Isle of Man*** [44]
~ After Baby is three months old, he can be given a coldwater sponge within a warm bath. Gradually lower the temperature until at ten months old, Baby can be sponged with quite cold water within a warm bath. This strengthens his constitution and makes him less susceptible to cold. No completely cold baths should be given until the child is four. ***Edwardian UK*** [27]
~ The colder the Bath the better...it's necessary for hardening the child to life's cruelties.
~ Wash the child's feet every day in cold water to toughen him up. Then make him sit with wet feet. ***18th Century USA***
~ Put a child to bed wrapped in cold wet towels to toughen him up. ***Slovenia***
~ Whoever bathes in cold water on Easter day, keeps well the whole year. ***Germany*** [1]
~ A newborn can't be washed on a Friday. ***Turkey***
~ A baby washed on Friday is robbed of his rest. ***Germany*** [1]
~ Don't wash Baby's hair on a Sunday if you wish him to be successful in life. ***Greece***

DRESSING BABY

~ For good luck throughout the year, dress Baby in new clothes at Easter.
~ All flannel clothing aired by the window and then by the fire, will often last Baby one week. ***Edwardian UK*** [27]
~ Only Baby's face and hands should be exposed to the air. All internal organs and large skin surfaces must be kept covered up. ***Edwardian UK*** [27]
~ To measure a child for clothes in his first year, spoils his figure. ***Germany*** [1]
~ Don't allow the front part of Baby's head to be exposed to the sun, as it will surely irritate his brain so congestion and fits will ensue. A cabbage leaf placed under Baby's hat will help protect against the sun's rays. ***Edwardian*** [27]
~ A knitted belt to reach from the hips to the armpits and to which the nappy can be pinned, will avert the risks of Baby catching the chill that leads to constipation and diarrhoea. In older children, a large expanse of thigh and leg left uncovered also leads to constipation and diarrhoea, therefore the child must wear flannel drawers fitting closely just above the knees. ***Edwardian*** [27]
~ Make older babies wear clothes and shoes so thin they leak and let in water to toughen them up. ***18th Century USA***
~ When Baby is a little older, a belt must be worn to protect his abdominal organs. ***Edwardian UK*** [27]

~ Mending a hem or button while Baby is still wearing the damaged garment brings misfortune. ***Russia***
~ Put red pepper in Baby's shoes to keep him out of trouble.
~ Never put new shoes on a table. ***UK***
~ If red shoes are put on a child under a year old, he'll never see blood. ***Germany*** [1]
~ As many steps as a child takes in one shoe, so many whippings will he receive.
~ Never let a child walk in one shoe, as it will cause either his mother or father to die. ***Belize & Russia***
~ If Baby's shoes are placed on the wrong feet, he'll have an accident with one of his feet.
~ It's luckier to put on both stockings first, and then shoes. ***German Pennsylvania***
~ When putting on, or taking off Baby's shoes, always start with the right one first or it causes bad luck and Baby may die early.

CUTTING BABY'S NAILS

~ Let the nail cuttings fall on an open Bible, so Baby grows up honest. ***UK***
~ Cutting nails with clippers will cause poor eyesight.
~ Baby's nails must never be cut during his first month of life. ***Vietnam***
~ Cutting a baby's nails with scissors before he's one year's old will make him a thief. ***Newfoundland, Cornwall UK & Wolof People Senegal***
~ Nails should be bitten, not cut, for the same time. ***Europe***
~ Nails should be cut when the moon is on the increase to make them grow strong. Clipping fingernails in the dark of the moon will bring bad luck.
~ Nails can't be cut at nights (*Turkey, Madagascar, Vietnam & Java*), for fear of angering evil spirits (*India*), or bringing a visit from a ghost. (*China*)
~ It's bad luck to cut fingernails on a Friday or Sunday.
~ Never trim fingernails on Sunday as you'll see blood before Monday or evil stories will be told about you throughout the week. 'Sunday's horn goes to the devil on Monday morn.' ***UK***
~ Cutting nails on Holy Innocents Day is unlucky.
~ Cut Baby's nails on Sunday, or Friday, to prevent toothache. ***German Pennsylvania***
~ Fingernails and toenails aren't cut together or Baby will face one sorrowful act and one joyful event. ***Turkey***
~ Start clipping the nail of the little finger on the right hand, finishing with the thumb. ***Morocco***[20]
~ You always ought to begin with the forefinger of the right hand, as it's the most honourable of all the digits. ***Yemen***[20]
~ According to Mohammed, the order is remembered by the word *Khawabis*

which indicates the initials of the names of the five fingers of the hand. First one is to attend to the *Khansar* (little finger), then the *Wasti* (middle finger), then the *Abham* (thumb), then the *Binsar* (ring finger), and last of all to the *Sababa* (index finger). ***Islamic***[20]

'Cut them on Monday, you cut them for health;
cut them on Tuesday, you cut them for wealth;
cut them on Wednesday, you cut them for news;
cut them on Thursday, a new pair of shoes;
cut them on Friday, you cut them for sorrow;
cut them on Saturday, see your true love tomorrow;
cut them on Sunday, the devil will be with you all the week.'

'Cut your nails in Monday, cut them for news; (of success)
Cut them on Tuesday for a new pair of shoes;
Cut them on Wednesday, cut them for health;
Cut them for Thursday, cut them for wealth;
Cut them on Friday, a sweetheart to know; (also a good way to avoid neuralgia)
Cut them on Saturday, a journey to go;
Cut them on Sunday, you cut them for evil,
For all the next week you'll be ruled by the Devil.'

'Monday for news.
Tuesday for shoes.
Wednesday for wealth.
Thursday for health.
Friday for woe.
Saturday for a journey to go.
Sunday for evil.'

(For disposal of nail clippings see page 189)

BABY'S HAIR

~ If Baby is wrapt in fur when born, he'll have curly hair. ***Germany***[1]
~ The colour of Baby's hair at birth is a true reflection of what it shall be like in adulthood. ***Edwardian UK***[27]
~ During dog days, if rain falls on Baby's head, look out for baldness, or headache. ***German Pennsylvania USA***
~ If Baby's hair is cut, the child will get an elflock. ***Jewish***
~ If you shave Baby's head bald, his hair will grow back thicker. ***Russia***

~ A spirit called 'khuan' dwells in the human head, of which it's the guardian spirit. The spirit must be carefully protected from injury of every kind; hence the act of shaving or cutting the hair is accompanied with many ceremonies. ***Siam*** [14]
~ A comb picked up with its teeth facing the body is bad luck. ***Japan***
~ Hair will grow better if kept short for the first three years. ***Edwardian UK*** [27]
~ Hair, a symbol of fertility, increases its potency when in touch with water. Sinhalese parents cut a small tuft of the newborn's hair and throw it into a river, so it mixes in water, and brings prosperity to the child. Since hair is used in black magic to bring harm, throwing the hair into water also signifies the destruction of evil that might affect the child in later life. ***Sri Lanka***
~ If Baby get sick a lot, shave his head and leave only the middle part. ***Thailand***
~ Keeping a tuft of hair on the top of the head brings Baby long life. The tuft helps protect the vital part of the head called Adhipathi ('overload'). Any injury to this part of the skull can cause sudden death. ***Hindi***
~ When hair is cut to rid it of vermin, some locks are allowed to remain on the crown of the head as a refuge for one of Baby's souls. ***The Toradjas People Indonesia*** [14]
~ The first hair which a child gets isn't his own, and if not cut off will make him weak and ill. Therefore, when Baby is about a month old, his hair is cut in a ceremony. Each of the friends invited to the ceremony snips off a little of Baby's hair and drops it into a coconut shell full of water. Afterwards, Dad takes the hair and packs it into a little bag made of leaves, which he fastens to the top of a palm tree. Then he gives the leaves of the palm a good shaking, climbs down, and goes home without speaking to anyone. ***Island of Rotti near Timor*** [20]
~ Baby's hair mustn't be cut during the first month of life (*Vietnam*), until he's baptised (*Greek Orthodox*), until he begins to crawl or walk (*Indian Tribes Guyana*[21]), or until he's at least one. Otherwise, Baby's hair will be thin or his development will be held up. There's a saying, 'cutting before one is cutting off a tongue.' (*Russia*)
~ It's bad luck to cut a child's hair before he turns one as he'll lose his strength. If the hair becomes too long, bite it off instead of cutting. ***Poland, UK & Germany***
~ Don't even comb Baby's hair until he's a year old. ***India***
~ Cutting a child's hair when he's too young diminishes his eyesight. ***Slavic***
~ The longer Baby's hair is allowed to grow without being cut, the more intelligent he will be. ***French Canada***
~ Hair wasn't cut before the child was seven in some provinces, lest it hinder his development. ***Russia***

~ It's bad luck to cut hair when a family member's health is in danger. ***Russia***
~ It's good luck to cut hair during a storm.
~ Haircutting was viewed as dangerous. The most sacred day of the year was that appointed for haircutting. A spell was uttered to avert thunder and lightning. ***New Zealand*** [14]
~ The chief always ate a man as precaution when he had his hair cut. ***Namosi: Fiji*** [14]
~ Haircuts must be done by the new moon only; otherwise, the hair can't grow again. ***France*** [1]
~ Cut hair on a waxing moon for growth, on a waning moon to discourage growth. ***Cornwall UK*** [12]
~ 'Friday's hair…goes to the devil on Monday morn.'
~ The 'chudakarma' ceremony is normally performed in Baby's thirteenth month. Shaving and cutting the hair and nails at this ceremony removes impurities and gives Baby lightness, long life, prosperity, bravery and health and beauty. ***Hindi***

DISPOSAL OF HAIR & NAIL CLIPPINGS

~ The first cut hair was hidden under the house or stuck into the tie beam. ***Russia***
~ The first hair cut from a boy is put in his father's pocket to increase his fortune.
~ The first lock of hair is saved and hidden in a safe place to bring luck and a long life.
~ When a child's topknot has been cut with great ceremony, the short hairs are put into a little vessel made of plantain leaves and set adrift on the nearest river. As the hair floats away, all that is harmful in the child's disposition departs with it. The long hairs are kept until the child makes a pilgrimage to the Holy Footprint of Buddha on the sacred hill at Prabat. It's then presented to the priests, who make them into brushes with which they sweep the Footprint. ***Siam*** [14]
~ Hang the cut hair on a tree growing on or near the grave of a wonderworking saint; to rid Baby of headache or guard against it. ***Morocco***
~ Great care must be taken in disposing of clippings, especially the first clippings, as Baby can suffer if clippings are harmed as they are still part of his body even when severed. ***Malaysia*** [20]
~ If nail trimmings are thrown on the ground, Satan makes use of them. If they're trodden on, Baby could become very ill. ***Algeria*** [20]
~ Anyone walking over Baby's nail clippings will dislike Baby. ***Germany*** [1]
~ If hair clippings aren't put in a cool spot, Baby will suffer. ***Indonesia***
~ If hair or nail clippings are disturbed by animals, Baby will get sick. ***Yukon Indians: Alaska***

~ It's unlucky for Baby if water is poured on his clippings. ***Algeria*** [20]
~ If hair is carried away by the wind, Baby will suffer from giddiness. ***Tunisia***
~ If hair clippings are carried away by a bird, Baby's hair will fall out. (*Germany*[1]) If birds or mice build their nests with Baby's hair, Baby will suffer from headache or get a boil on his head. (*UK*) Hair should be burnt; otherwise, birds might make a nest of the hair, weaving tightly, so Baby would have difficulty rising on the last day. (*Cornwall UK*)
~ Hair clippings left to fly about make the pathway to heaven difficult. ***Java*** [20]
~ Hair, skin and nails make powerful magical potions which can be used against their former owners. You shouldn't throw hair in the rubbish as someone could pick it up and bring harm to Baby. ***Japan***
~ Hair clippings mustn't be thrown on the streets or witches could cast a spell on it. ***France***[1]
~ Witches use cut or combed out hair to make hailstones or thunderstorms with. ***Austria***[14]
~ To spit on cut hair before throwing it away, is thought in some parts of Europe sufficient to prevent its use by witches. [19]
~ It's wicked to throw nail clippings away. They should be buried or burned. ***Jewish***
~ Bury nail clippings under the eaves on the north side of the house. ***German Pennsylvania***
~ Bury the first nail clippings under an ash tree so the child will be a fine singer. ***Northumberland UK***
~ Burn toenail clippings for luck. ***UK***
~ Hair is buried in a bag under the threshold (*Danzig Austria*[14]), under an elder bush tree three days before the new moon (*Germany*[14]), in some remote place where they won't be trodden upon (*Morocco*), or in a spot where neither sun nor moon can shine on it. (*Swabia Germany*[14])
~ If toenail cuttings are thrown onto the ground, the owner will be forced to pick them up when he dies.
~ The Armenians hide their cut hair and nails and extracted teeth in 'holy' places, such as a crack in the church wall, or a hollow tree, as all these severed portions of themselves will be needed at the Resurrection. Those who have not safely stowed them away will have to hunt about for them on the great day. [14]
~ The Incas took extreme care to preserve their clippings, placing them in holes in the walls as their souls must rise out of the tombs with all that belonged to their bodies. They were careful also to spit in only one place.' [14]
~ In Java, clippings are wrapped up and buried while saying, 'Abide here until I die and when I die follow me.' [20] In Iraq, clippings are preserved in bottles, and in Turkey, they're carefully stowed in the cracks of walls or floorboards.
~ The hairs of the head are all numbered by the Almighty, and one will have to

account for them on the Day of Judgment. For this reason, hair was stuffed away in the thatch of the cottages. ***Drumconrath Ireland*** [14]

~ During the last days, Satan will appear on earth riding a mule. Every hair on the mule's body is a tuned string. By his music … all the people on earth are tempted to follow Satan. Great horns grow out on their heads, so they can never return through their doors. The faithful Mohammedan has, however, carefully collected his nail clippings, and placed them under the doors' threshold, where they have formed a hedge, to prevent the household from running after Satan. ***Chinese Turkestan*** [20]

~ Owls (commonly thought of as witch birds) enter the house at night to gather human fingernails. ***Inner Mongolia***

BABIES AND MIRRORS

~ A child must not be held before a mirror; else a second child will be born within the year. ***Jewish***

~ It's unlucky for a baby to see his reflection before he is six months old (*UK*) or until he cuts his first tooth. (*Jewish*)

~ If a Baby under one year's old looks in a mirror, he'll have bad dreams (*Kyrgyzstan*), the soul will be sacred out of his body (*Slavic*), he'll become dumb (*India*), grow up vain (*Germany*), or die. (*India*)

Baby Lore

CHAPTER 23
BELIEFS, REMEDIES & CHARMS FOR BABY'S AILMENTS

> NB. Extreme care must be taken if deciding to test out any of these theories. While some beliefs may be harmless fun, or even work, *some* are dangerous to Baby's Health. Always consult a qualified medical practitioner if in *any* doubt.

~ Allowing Baby to suck his fingers causes hairy knuckles.
~ If the fontanelle is sunken, tap Baby's feet or the roof of his mouth to move his brain back up.
~ Anyone with an ailment or deformity must have been in or near the woods after dark and been pinched by a fairy. *Newfoundland*
~ Castor oil once a month keeps children healthy. *Italy*
~ Cover Baby's stomach so he doesn't get sick. *China*
~ Put bicarbonate of soda paste or egg-white on nappy rash.
~ Coral beads are said to change colour indicating whether the wearer is ill or well. *Cornwall UK*
~ The nursery should be high up, south or west-facing and well ventilated. The nursery must be aired for several hours each day, as must the bed linen, and then warmed up by a fire to 60 degrees Fahrenheit before Baby is returned to it. Air becomes poisonous if the nursery isn't aired, and many babies have lost their frail little lives from lack of this knowledge. To ensure freshness, allow 1000 cubic feet of space per person who occupies the room (excluding furniture). *Edwardian UK* [27]
~ If Baby's testes don't come down, place a heated cucumber or leaf over them. *Thailand*
~ If Baby gets sick, someone is jealous of the baby or the family. The parents must take Baby to a Cuededa (healer) who chants after wrapping up Baby's belly as he's believed to have an upside-down stomach. *Portugal*
~ The hand of a suicide's corpse was used as a charm to cure illnesses, by placing on the afflicted spot. Going to be touched by one newly hung on the gallows also cures many diseases. *Cornwall UK* [12]
~ Mistletoe which grows on an oak is a remedy for every childhood disease and ailment. It must not be cut in the usual way but be caught as it falls to the ground (*Switzerland* [14]), or must be shot down out of the oak or knocked down with stones. (*Sweden & Wales*)
~ For mesenteric illnesses, children were dipped three times in Chapell Uny well against the sun, then dragged around the well three times on the grass in

the same direction. ***Cornwall UK*** [12]

~ For Water on the Brain: Cover the head well with wool, then place oilskin over it, and the water will be drawn up out of the head. When the wool is saturated the brain will be free and the child cured. ***Ireland*** [15]

~ A trout or other small live fish, passed through the mouth of a slobbering baby, and then returned alive to the stream works wonders. ***German Pennsylvania USA***

~ If Baby is licked by a dog, he'll be a quick healer.

~ For snakebite, catch a toad and tie it to the wound. If the toad dies, repeat the operation until the toad remains alive. ***German Pennsylvania USA***

~ The Thordall Insect got safe in a bottle and kept prisoner till it dies, makes the disease go away from the patient. ***Ireland*** [15]

~ When a child dwindles, tie a red silk thread around his neck, then catch a mouse, pass the thread with a needle through its skin over the backbone, and let it go. The mouse wastes, and the child picks up. ***Germany*** [1]

~ Children of all diseases were carried to the seashore and passed through a cleft of rock at Perranzabalo. ***Cornwall UK*** [12]

~ A sick child gets better if his godfather carries him three times up and down the room. ***Germany***

~ Don't pay the doctor, at least in full, if you would avoid sickness in the family. ***German Pennsylvania USA***

~ A Baby's head should be stroked often so it becomes nicely rounded. ***China***

~ Massage Baby's arms and legs with boiled rice water to prevent bowlegs and cocked arm. ***Thailand***

~ Go before sunrise on May Day to collect dew from the churchyard that will heal all manner of illnesses. ***Cornwall UK*** [12]

~ All holy water is good for healing, or preventing witchcraft or spirits. ***UK***

~ 'When children are sick, and languish long in their malady, so they waste away, they are taken away (at least in substance) by Fairies, and only the shadow left with them; so, at a particular season in summer, parents leave their child out all night by themselves, near Therdy Hill in Inverness-shire while watching at a distance, and this they imagine will either 'end or mend them'; they say many more do recover than don't.' ***Scotland*** [58]

~ 'In a consumptive disease, the fairies steal away the soul, and put a fairy's soul in place of it. A practice, apparently of druidical origin, is used to avert this danger. In the increase of the March moon, withes of oak and ivy are cut, and twisted into wreaths or circles, which they preserve until the next March. After that period, when persons are consumptive, or children hectic, they cause them to pass thrice through these circles.' ***East Coast of Scotland*** [58]

~ When children are pining away, they are fairy struck; and the juice of twelve leaves of foxglove should be given as a remedy. ***Ireland***

~ The rosary is widely used for the cure of the sick and is used for the cure of 'retention of urine' in children. It's put on Baby's neck or laid on the roof in the starlight to catch the dew, then washed and the water given to Baby to drink. *Egypt* [20]
The rosary is used to decide what medicine should be taken, what doctor should be called, whether his advice should be followed, etc. *Iraq* [20]
~ With the rosary in the hand, read any chapter from the Koran up to the fifteenth verse, as this verse always contains a word of talismanic power. *Indonesia* [20]
~ Potina is the Roman Goddess of Children's medicine and the safe drinking ability of children.

PATRON SAINTS

Patron Saints of sick children; Beuno, Clement I, Hugh of Lincoln, Ubaldus Baldassini
Patron Saints of childhood diseases: Aldegundis, Pharaildis
Patron Saint of Nurses; Agatha, Alexius, Camillus of Lellis, Catherine of Alexandria, Catherine of Siena, John of God, Margaret of Antioch, Raphael the Archangel
Patron Saint of Backward Children; Hilary of Poitiers
Patron Saints of the Disabled; Alphais, Angela Merici, Gerard of Aurillac, Germaine Cousin, Giles, Henry II, Lutgardis, Margaret of Castello, Seraphina, Servatus, Servulus
Patron Saint of Long Life; Peter the Apostle

SPECIFIC TREATMENTS A~Z

- **BIRTHMARKS, FRECKLES AND OTHER BLEMISHES**

~ To make a birthmark disappear, apply saliva (*Celtic*), the dew of May morning (*Cornwall UK*), rub it with a duck's foot (*Germany*), or the hand of a corpse and it will disappear at the same rate as the corpse decomposes (*Europe & USA*) Alternately, touch it with your tongue for nine mornings and it will fade away.
~ If it rains on Baby while there is a rainbow, he'll get freckles. Raindrops on a child under a year will also cause freckles. To got rid of them, requires rising early in the morning of a certain day, and washing the face with dew. *German Pennsylvania*
~ On meeting a funeral, take some of the clay from under the feet of the pallbearers and apply it to the blemish, wishing strongly at the same time that it may disappear; and so it will. *Ireland* [15]

- **BLEEDING**

~ Drinking powdered coral is very good for nosebleeds.
~ For nosebleeds, get Baby to chew newspaper (*German Pennsylvania*), tie lengths of red thread around Baby's neck (*Pagan*), place a cold key down his

back (*UK*), or place a brown paper bag or dime under his tongue. (*African American*)

~ Some of the blood from the nose is covered with earth, and the following verse repeated;
'Pçuvus, I give to thee,
Pçuvus, oh take from me,
Give it to thy child,
it's very warm,
Take it quickly!' ***Romany Gypsy***[7]

~ Some miners were able to charm illnesses from the child. To stop bleeding, erysipelas, ringworms, pains and ulcers, they said;
'Christ was born at Bethlehem
Baptised in the River Jordan
The river stood so shall thy blood (name of baby)
In the Name of the Father, Son and Holy Ghost.' ***Cornwall UK***[12]

- **BONE PROBLEMS**

~ For rickets or bone problems, Baby was passed 'three times three times' against the sun through a young ash tree that had been spilt vertically downwards. The tree was bound back together and if it survived, Baby regained health and strength. For other diseases, the naked child was passed through nine times headfirst. A variation was Mum and Baby passed through three times, and the child was washed for three successive mornings in the dew from the charmed ash. ***Cornwall UK***[12]

~ The Roman God Ossipaga hardened the bones of the infant

~ Treat the child with a diet of raw meat juice, cream and cod liver oil. ***Edwardian UK***[27]

~ Bath rickety children on the first three Wednesdays in May at one of the holy Wells. ***Cornwall UK***[12]

- **CANCER**

~ Stroke a tumour with the hand of a corpse, and it will disappear with the decomposition of the corpse. Also a toad, if applied to cancer, will suck out the poison and thus cause a cure. ***German Pennsylvania***

- **CHICKEN POX**

~ Calamine lotion, oatmeal in a bath or paste, cornflower and water, baking soda and Vaseline, lemon juice, flour scorched in skillet, olive oil to prevent drying and scarring, warm sardine grease, and catnip tea are all said to be remedies. ***African American***

~ Blowing cigarette smoke on some milk given on a spoon to the child is a cure. ***African American***

~ Asafoetida worn in a bag around the child's neck acts as a charm. ***USA***

- **COLDS/COUGHS/CHEST**

~ The touch of a piebald horse cures coughs and colds. Even a piebald horse pawing before the door helps. *Ireland* [15]

~ Alternately, wear an amber bead necklace (*UK*), skunk oil in a bag around the neck (*African American*), a mustard poultice (*Italy*), a linseed poultice with mustard (*Edwardian UK*) or an onion (*African American*). Also try breathing on Baby's head, tapping his forehead with an onion (*Thailand*), or giving him juice from a baked onion.

~ Tie a red string around Baby's throat and then pass him seven times under and over a donkey. *Ireland* [15]

~ To cure a cough: take a hair from the child's head, put it between two slices of buttered bread, feed it to a dog, and say, 'Eat well, you hound, may you be sick and (name of baby) be sound.' *UK*

~ In Sunderland, they shaved the Baby's crown and hung the hair upon a bush so birds carrying the hair to their nests carried away the child's cough with it.

~ Nine hairs from a black cat's tail, chopped up and soaked in water which is then swallowed, will relieve coughs. *Ireland* [15]

~ Cure for chin cough; a griddle cake made of meal, to be given of love or of charity, but not for begging; not bought or made; a cake given freely, with a prayer and a blessing; and from the breakfast of a man and his wife who had the same name before marriage; this is the cure. *Ireland* [15]

~ A sheep's lung applied to the feet of a pneumonia sufferer draws the disease downward into itself. *UK*

~ Letting Baby run naked around the nursery each day will be a daily treat, and lessen his liability to catch cold. *Edwardian UK* [27]

~ A child suffering with any chest disease must not talk. *Edwardian UK* [27]

~ Make a child vomit to bring up the phlegm of bronchitis. *Edwardian UK* [27]

~ Pleurisy is believed to be caused by the attachment of the liver to the ribs; the cure being to break this adhesion by stretching the body. The disease is commonly known as livergrown: literally; grown fast.[65]

~ Lay a livergrown child on a doorsill and measure him. When the child has outgrown this measure the complaint will also be forgotten. *German Pennsylvania*

~ If a child was livergrown, or seemed to have a spell, he was put three times through a horse collar taken from a horse still warm. Good also for wind, colic, or gripes. Alternately, pass the child beneath a table to an assistant. *German Pennsylvania* [65]

~ Patron Saints against coughs; Blaise, Quentin, Walburga

~ Patron Saint of lungs, chest, respiratory problems; Bernadine of Siena

- **CONVULSIONS & FITS**

~ To treat convulsions, give Baby a hot bath and castor oil (*Edwardian UK* [27]).

lay a horseshoe under Baby's pillow (***Germany*** [1]), or place under the cradle of Baby's hair and nail clippings tied up in a linen cloth. *(Ireland)*
~ The use of coral helps the children of the 'falling evil' (epilepsy). ***UK***
~ Seizures in children can be treated with a broth made from Owl eyes (*India*) or by eating the heart of a rattlesnake. (*German Pennsylvania*)
~ Patron Saints of convulsive children; Guy of Anderlecht, John the Baptist, Scholastica

- **CRADLE CAP**

~ To relieve cradle cap, rub a wet nappy on Baby's head, or massage Vitamin E cream, Almond Oil, Baby Oil or butter onto his scalp.
~ Put Vaseline on the scalp at night, and then wash off in the morning. ***Edwardian UK*** [27]

- **CROUP**

~ Treat children with croup with a hot bath with mustard and make the child vomit to shorten the attack. ***Edwardian UK*** [27]
~ A common remedy for croup is to administer a mixture of goose grease and molasses to induce vomiting. Alternately, mix urine and goose grease and administer internally, and also rub some of the mixture over the breast and throat. ***Pennsylvania***
~ Make a poultice of grated pokeroot and vinegar and apply to Baby's feet, or mix juice from three to five boiled onions with honey and give to the child. ***Pennsylvania***
~ A pearl shell bearing the image of Saint Francis of Assisi worn by children brings a cure for croup. ***Italy*** [7]

- **EARS**

~ To cure earache, blow cigarette smoke in Baby's ears, insert warmed drops of cod liver oil, camphor oil, or sweet oil into the ear, or put a warm towel, warm ashes, or a warm pebble in the ear to draw moisture out. ***African American***
~ Baby's own urine treats earache. ***Pennsylvania USA***
~ Patron Saints of against earaches; Cornelius, Polycarp of Smyrna
~ Patron Saints of the deaf; Cadoc of Llancarvan, Drogo, Francis de Sales, Meriadoc, Ouen

- **EYES**

~ The whilks on child's eyelids are cured by passing a black cat's tail (preferably a Tom Cat's) nine times over the eyelid. ***Cornwall UK*** [12]
~ Sore eyes can be relieved by a few drops of breast milk. ***Belize & Celtic***
~ A son who never knew his father is able to melt wens, by touching them three mornings in a row, before breaking his fast and saying a few prayers. ***France***[1]
~ Club moss is good for the eyes. On the 3rd day of the moon when the thin

crescent is seen for the first time, show the moon the knife to cut the moss and say,
'As Christ healed the issue of blood
Do thou cut, what thou cutest for good.'
At sundown, wash your hands and while kneeling cut the club moss. Wrap it in a white cloth, and boil this in water taken from the spring nearest its place of growth. This can be made into an ointment or fomentation for eye problems. (NB. If you tell other people this particular charm, you will lose the personal power to do it yourself.) ***Cornwall UK*** [12]

~ For weak wyes, a decoction of boiled down daisies is an excellent wash, to be used constantly. ***Ireland*** [15]

~ Don't look at Baby from behind or you'll cross his eyes. ***Belize***

~ When Baby is lying down and looks up towards the head of the crib, there's a tendency for his eyes to get crossed. When this happens, get a bright coloured piece of string, wet it, and place it across the bridge of his nose. Baby will then keep his eyes straight. ***Spain***

~ **Roman Catholic Patron Saints of Eyes, Eye Diseases and Problems:** Aloysius Gonzaga, Augustine of Hippo, Clare of Assisi, Cyriacus of Iconium, Erhard of Regensburg, Herve, Leodegarius, Lucy of Syracuse, Odilia, Raphael the Archangel, Symphorian of Autun

~ **Patron Saints of the Blind:** Catald, Cosmas, Damian, Dunstan, Lawrence the Illiuminator, Leodegarius, Lucy, Lutgardis, Odilia, Parasceva, Raphael the Archangel, Thomas the Apostle

- **FEVER**

~ To banish convulsive fevers, write the following letters on a piece of white paper, sew it on a piece of linen or muslin, and bang it around Baby's neck until the fever goes:
A b a x a C a t a b a x
A b a x a C a t a b a x
A b a x a C a t a b a
A b a x a C a t a b
A b a x a C a t a
A b a x a C a t
A b a x a C a
A b a x a C
A b a x a
A b a x
A b a
A b ***German Pennsylvania*** [24]

~ To cure fever, put a swallow's nest under Baby's pillow (*Germany¹*), give Baby only milk (*Edwardian UK,*) feed him the juice of twelve leaves of

foxglove (*Ireland*), or hailstones to eat as a preventative cure (*German Pennsylvania*).
~ To banish a fever, write the following words upon a paper and wrap it up in knot-grass, and then tie it upon the child's body: '*Potmat sineat, Potmat sineat, Potmat sineat.*'
~ Place Baby on a sandy shore when the tide is coming in and the retreating waves will carry away the disease and leave him well. ***Ireland*** [15]
~ Take three bits of stolen bread, spit in two nutshells, and write this note, 'Cow, will you go to your stall, Fever go you to the wall.' ***France*** [1]
~ The sick child must not eat pork, drink milk, or cross running water, for nine days ***German Pennsylvania*** [24]
~ The first bucket pulled from a well at midnight, cures fever. Near Nogent-le-Rotrou there is a spring famous for its curing virtues during the whole of Saint John's Night. Men and women get into its waters and wash themselves: the ceremony isn't disturbed by any idea of indecency. ***France*** [1]
~ Earwax applied on fever blisters works.

- **HEAD PROBLEMS**

~ If there's pain in one side of Baby's head, Mum should look at the rays of the setting sun, rubbing the affected portion with a few blades of grass, while muttering an incantation three times.
~ To be free from headache, rub the forehead with a piece of iron or stone. ***Slavic***
~ To cure headache, the 'taleb' takes hold of the patient's head with the first finger and thumb across the brow and gently blow upon his face until the pain has disappeared. ***Algeria*** [20]
~ When a child bumps his head, the swelling is pressed with a knife blade, and the following spell is muttered three, seven, or nine times, according to the gravity of the injury:
'Be thou, be thou, be thou weak (i.e., soft)
And very soon perish!
Go thou into the earth,
May I see thee never more
Bring knives, knives,
Give (i.e., put) into the earth.'
Then the knife is stuck three, seven, or nine times into the earth. ***Romany*** [7]

- **HICCUPS**

~ Have Baby wear red to protect from hiccups.
~ Get Baby to smell dill. ***UK***
~ Stick to Baby's forehead a tiny piece of wet paper (*Spain*), or a thread moistened with saliva (*Philippines*)
~ Administer castor oil to get rid of hiccups. ***USA***

~ When anyone has hiccups they're believed to be owned by the devil.
~ When children have hiccups their heart is growing (*Germany*[1]) or someone is talking or thinking about them. (*India*)
~ When anyone hiccups, it is etiquette to say, 'You stole something from me,' to bring good luck. ***Turkestan*** [3]

- **INFECTION/WOUNDS**

~ A bunch of mint tied round the wrist keeps off infection and disease. ***Ireland***
~ Sterilise a wound by sucking it with your mouth; or urinate on it. ***German Pennsylvania***
~ If Baby has a sore or cut, don't give him any protein to eat to prevent infection. ***Thailand***
~ Patron Saint of Bacterial Disease and Infection: Agrippina

- **INFLAMMATION**

~ To reduce inflammation, poultice it with warm cow dung, or other semi-liquid dung. ***German Pennsylvania***
~ Patron Saint against inflammatory diseases: Benedict

- **KIDNEYS**

~ Kidney Disease may be cured by using goat titrine. ***German Pennsylvania***
~ Bicarbonate of soda treats urine infections. ***Edwardian UK*** [27]
~ **Patron Saints of Kidney Disease**; Benedict, Drogo, Margaret of Antioch, Ursus of Ravenna
~ **Patron Saint of Jaundice**; Odilo

- **MEASLES**

~ This is to be repeated three times, kneeling at a cross, for three mornings before sunrise, and the child will be cured by the following Sunday .
'The child has the measles,' said John the Baptist.
'The time is short till he is well,' said the Son of God.
'When?' said John the Baptist.
'Sunday morning, before sunrise,' said the Son of God. ***Ireland*** [15]

- **MUMPS**

~ Take Baby into a pigsty, and rub the swollen neck a certain odd number of times on the front edge of the hog trough. ***German Pennsylvania***

- **NAVEL**

~ If Baby has a large navel, Dad must push his big toe into it when he returns from a long journey and it will return to normal. ***Guyana***
~ Take a beggar's staff from a beggar silently, and press the navel with it crosswise to cure an enlarged navel. ***Germany*** [1]
~ Place a silver dollar on Baby's belly button to prevent an 'outie'. ***Hispanic***
~ Spit on the naval frequently, so the cord will drop off sooner. ***Thailand***

- **RASHES, BRUISES & BURNS**

~ To cure a rash, get a piece of wood out of a millwheel, set it alight, and smoke the swathings with it; then wash Baby with water bounding off the millwheel. What is left of the wood shall be thrown into running water. ***Germany*** [1]

~ Apply raw beef or eau de cologne with Vaseline to bruises. For mild scalds, use a strong solution of bicarbonate of soda applied with rags. For bad burns apply Vaseline and Eucalyptus oil or Olive oil and lime water. ***Edwardian*** [27]

~ Lard, mayonnaise, toothpaste, mustard, and ashes from a fireplace all treat burns. ***African American***

~ For a scald or burn, dock or bramble leaves wetted with spring water are placed on the afflicted area and then angels are invoked from the east.

'There came three angels out of the east,
One brought fire and two brought frost;
Our fire and in frost,
In the Name of the Father, Son and Holy Ghost, ame.n' ***Cornwall UK*** [12]

~ Ringworm infections are cured by rubbing a green walnut on the infection.

~ Lice cause eczema. ***Edwardian UK*** [27]

~ For a nettle sting get a dock leaf and chant; 'Out nettle, in dock, Docks shall have new smock' ***Cornwall UK*** [12]

~ Rub Baby on pigs' litter to stop hives. ***German Pennsylvania***

~ **Patron Saints of Skin Diseases, Rashes, Eczema:** Anthony the Abbott, George, Marculf, Peregrine Laziosi, Roch

- **SPRAINS**

~ The 'wresting thread' is a black woollen thread, on which are cast nine knots. It's tied round a sprained limb while the one who is applying the remedy whispers, so as not to be heard by even the patient:

'The Lord rade,
And the foal slade;
He lighted.
And he righted.
Set joint to joint,
Bone to bone,
And sinew to sinew.
Heal in the Holy Ghost's Name!' ***Shetland and Orkney Islands*** [66]

- **STOMACH**

~ A 5-8 month old baby will get diarrhoea because his body is stretching. ***Thailand***

~ A bunch of mint tied round the waist is a sure remedy for stomach disorders. ***Ireland***

~ To put a clean shirt on Baby on a Friday is good for the gripes. ***Germany*** [1]

~ The fifth son, born in a row, cures spleen diseases by mere repeated touch. ***France*** [1]

~ For a one-month-old baby, ten drops of brandy diluted in three times water is given every four hours to treat vomiting and diarrhoea. For a three-month-old, 20 to 30 drops of brandy can be given. Flatulence is relieved by bicarbonate of soda. ***Edwardian UK*** [27]

~ If Baby has stomach pains, the hair of a black dog is burned to powder and kneaded with Mum's milk and some of Baby's faeces into a paste. This is put into a cloth and bound onto Baby's belly. When Baby falls asleep, a hole is bored in a tree and the paste put into it. The hole is then stopped up with a wooden plug, and while this is being done the following is repeated:-
'Depart from the belly, Live in the green! (tree)
Remain, remain thou here, I say, I say to thee!' ***4th Century Gypsy charm*** [7]

~ Massage Baby's tummy regularly with balm so his stomach skin thickens to protect his insides, and to lessen stomach ache. ***Thailand***

~ If Baby is crying inconsolably and his face is a bluish hue with twitching eyes and mouth and cold extremities, give him two and a half grams of bicarbonate of soda in a tablespoon of warm water, dill water or peppermint water and place him on his stomach over a hot water bottle. ***Edwardian UK*** [27]

~ A teaspoon of dill water, caraway water, anise water, or peppermint water all treat colic, flatulence and other stomach ailments. For constipation: Give one teaspoon of olive oil or half a teaspoon of cod liver oil twice a day. To treat diarrhoea, give Baby egg-white in water, brandy, a warm bath with a tablespoon of mustard and raw meat juice. After indigestion, vomiting or diarrhoea give Baby an egg-white in water for his next meal. ***Edwardian UK*** [27]

~ If Baby suffers from stomach pains, a bit of nail must be clipped from each of his fingers, mixed with dried chicken dung, and Baby exposed to its smoke while it's burned. ***Romany Gypsy*** [7]

~ For colic, give Baby Chamomile tea and massage his belly with oil. ***Russia***

~ To cure colic, stand the child on his head for quarter of an hour. ***Cornwall*** [12]

~ Wrap a blanket tightly around Baby's stomach and compress to treat colic.

~ Carrying a new baby three times around the house will protect him from colic.

~ Say the following, "I warn ye, ye colic fiends! There is one sitting in judgment, who speaketh: just or unjust. Therefore beware, ye colic fiends!' ***German Pennsylvania*** [24]

~ Patron Saint of Abdominal Pains, Colic; Agapitus, Charles Borromeo, Erasmus

~ Patron Saint of Bowel Disorders: Bonaventure

~ Patron Saint of Childhood intestinal diseases: Erasmus

- **THROAT**

~ A wolf's right paw, tied around the throat, eases the swelling caused by throat infections.

~ Use urine to wash out Baby's sore mouth and throat. *USA*
~ Dummy's/pacifiers cause adenoids. *Edwardian UK* [27]
~ Thick barley water or blackcurrant tea treats sore throat. *Edwardian UK* [27]

- **THRUSH**

~ A bag filled with thirteen sow bugs tied around a child's neck will cure thrush, or sores in the mouth.
~ Use a cloth dipped in fresh Baby urine to wipe off thrush. *Belize*
~ Thrush results from sour milk or dirty stuffy nurseries. Treat with three grain doses of bicarbonate of soda twice a day for a 4 month old. The mouth should be swabbed with a rag dipped in boracic acid after meals. Borax dissolved in glycerine and painted on the tongue also treats thrush. *Edwardian* [27]
~ Someone who's never seen their natural father can blow into Baby's mouth and cure thrush.

- **WHOOPING COUGH**

~ To cure whooping cough, give Baby marble dust scraped off from a tombstone in Tabiz (*Iraq*), milk stolen from a neighbour's cow (*Pennsylvania: USA*), or tie lengths of red thread loosely around Baby's neck. (*Pagan*)
~ Wrap a piece of bread in cloth and bury it for three days, before digging it up and giving it to Baby to eat. *Suffolk: UK*
~ Find a sheep to breath on Baby, or put a live trout into the child's mouth; then, while still alive, put the trout back into the stream. Some say you need to get the trout to breathe three times into Baby's mouth for the full cure. *German Pennsylvania*
~ A steaming kettle with carbolic lotion treats whooping cough. *Edwardian* [27]
~ Cut three small bunches of hair from the crown of the head of a child who has never seen his father; sew this hair up in an unbleached rag and hang it with an unbleached thread around the sick child's neck. *German Pennsylvania* [24]
~ Thrust the child having the whooping cough three times through a blackberry bush, without speaking or saying anything. The bush, however, must be grownfast at the two ends, and the child must be thrust through three times from the same side. *German Pennsylvania* [24]
~ A three year old female donkey was taken and Baby was drawn naked nine times over its back and under its belly. Three hairs from the donkey's back and belly were placed in three spoonfuls of the donkey's milk; the mixture was stood for three hours, and then given to Baby to drink in three doses. The belief was that Christ riding into Jerusalem made the donkey holy, and if any child touched where Jesus sat, they'd no longer be ill. *Cornwall UK* [12]
~ **Patron Saints against Whooping Cough:** Blaise, Winnoc

Notes

[1] Vide Grimm's 'Teutonic Mythology', translated into English and kindly used by permission of The Northvegr Foundation at www.norvegr.com
[2] Michelle Klein, 'A Time to Be Born,' The Jewish Publication Society, 2001
[3] Robert Mearns Lawrence, 'The Magic Of The Horseshoe with other Folklore Notes', Boston And New York, Houghton, Mifflin & Co., 1898
[4] Hermann Hochegger (Ed), 'Encyclopedia of Ritual Symbolics' (R. D. Congo). Topics: Abandon to Zither, Ceeba publications, Antenne d'Autriche. St. Gabriel, Mödling, 2004.
[5] Thomas Firminger Thiselton-Dyer, 'Folklore of Women as illustrated by legendary and traditionary tales, folk rhymes, proverbial sayings, superstitions etc' London: Elliot Stock, 1906
[6] Thanks to Sigurd Towrie at www.orkneyjar.com
[7] 'Gypsy Sorcery And Fortune Telling' by Charles Godfrey Leland 'Gypsy Sorcery And Fortune Telling', Late President of the Gypsy Lore Society, London: T Fisher Unwin, 1891
[8] Thanks to Ulf Holmberg of Ulfie's Forge, a master blacksmith who makes these and other wonderful items, see www.uffes-smedja.nu
[9] Sabine Baring-Gould, 'A Book Of Folklore', London: Collins' Clear Type Press, 1913
[10] Bronislaw Malinowski, 'Baloma; the Spirits of the Dead in the Trobriand Islands' Originally published in' The Journal of the Royal Anthropological Institute of Great Britain and Ireland', Volume 46, 1916
[11] Ruth Edna Kelley, 'The Book of Hallowe'en', Boston: Lothrop, Lee and Shepard Co., 1919
[12] Robert Hunt, 'The Drolls, Traditions and Superstitions of Old Cornwall (Popular Romances of the West of England)' 2nd ed. London: John Camden Hotten, 1871
[13] John Arnott MacCulloch, 'The Religion of the Ancient Celts' Edinburgh: T. & T. Clark, 1911
[14] Sir James George Frazer, 'The Golden Bough, A Study of Magic and Religion', Abridged Edition, 1922
[15] Lady Francesca Speranza Wilde, 'Ancient Legends, Mystic Charms, and Superstitions of Ireland' London: Ward & Downey, 1887
[16] Eli Edward Burriss, 'Taboo, Magic, Spirits: A Study of Primitive Elements in Roman Religion' New York, Macmillan Company, 1931
[17] De Gubernatis, 'Zoological Mythology,' ii. 58 quoted by Charles Godfrey Leland, 'Gypsy Sorcery and Fortune Telling'
[18] James Bonwick, 'Irish Druids And Old Irish Religions' London: Griffith, Farran, 1894
[19] Frederick Thomas Elworthy, 'The Evil Eye - An Account of this Ancient and Widespread Superstition' London: J. Murray; 1895
[20] Samuel M. Zwemer F.R.G.S. 'The Influence of Animism on Islam: An Account of Popular Superstitions'
[21] Walter E. Roth, 'An Inquiry into the Animism and Folklore of the Guyana Indians'

from the Thirtieth Annual Report of the Bureau of American Ethnology, 1908-1909, pp. 103-386, Washington D.C., 1915

[22] R. O. Winstedt, 'Shaman, Saiva and Sufi, A Study of the Evolution of Malay Magic', Constable & Company Ltd, 1925

[23] 'Sad Dar' Translated by E. W. West, from 'Sacred Books of the East, volume 24' Clarendon Press, 1885.

[24] John George Hohman, 'Pow-Wows', 1820

[25] Jacob Grimm quoted by Charles Godfrey Leland in 'Gypsy Sorcery And Fortune Telling'

[26] Micha F. Lindemans, Chief Editor of Encyclopaedia Mythica www.pantheon.org

[27] Mrs. J Langston Hewer, 'Our Baby for Mothers and Nurses', London: John Wright & Co, 1908

[28] James Bonwick, 'Irish Druids And Old Irish Religions' London: Griffith, Farran, 1894

[29] Pliny Earle Goddard, 'Hupa Texts,' University of California Publications in American Archeology and Ethnology, Vol. 1, No. 2, 1904

[30] Thomas Keightley 'The Fairy Mythology Illustrative of the Romance and Superstition of Various Countries.' 1870

[31] 'Drums and Shadows' Georgia Writer's Project, 1940, Mary Granger, District Supervisor

[32] Karl Lyncker, 'Deutsche Sagen und Sitten in hessischen Gauen' (Kassel: Verlag von Oswald Bertram, 1854), no. 71

[33] Karl Bartsch, 'Sagen, Märchen und Gebräuche aus Meklenburg '[Mecklenburg] (Vienna: Wilhelm Braumüller, 1879), vol. 1

[34] Adalbert Kuhn and Wilhelm Schwartz, 'Norddeutsche Sagen, Märchen und Gebräuche' (Leipzig: F. A. Brockhaus, 1848)

[35] Melville and Frances Herskovits, 'Suriname Folklore' p. 42, quoted in 'Drums and Shadows'

[36] Meek, 'Law and Authority in a Nigerian Tribe' pp. 290~91, quoted in 'Drums and Shadows'

[37] Melville and Frances Herskovits, 'Suriname Folklore' p. 42 quoted in 'Drums and Shadows'

[38] Nassau, 'Fetichism in West Africa, p. 206. Quoted in 'Drums and Shadows'

[39] Meek, 'Law and Authority in a Nigerian Tribe' p. 291 quoted in 'Drums and Shadows'

[40] Nassau, 'Fetichism in West Africa, p. 206. Quoted in 'Drums and Shadows'

[41] Eli Edward Burriss, 'Taboo, Magic, Spirits: A Study of Primitive Elements in Roman Religion' quoting Aelius Lampridius, Diadumenus Antoninus IV. 2.

[42] Thomas, 'Anthropological Report on the Ibo-Speaking Peoples of Nigeria,' I, pp. 10-11 quoted in 'Drums and Shadows'

[43] T. Sharper Knowlson, 'The Origins of Popular Superstitions and Customs,' 1910

[44] William Cashen, 'Manx Folk Lore' Douglas: G & L Johnson, 1912

[45] Francis Bacon, 'Works', London: 1740, iii. 187.

[46] Charles Godfrey Leland, 'Etruscan Roman Remains in Popular Tradition' London: T. Fisher Unwin, 1892
[47] Rev. Robert Hamill, 'Nassau Fetichism in West Africa' Charles Scribners & Son, 1904
[48] Edward Shortland, 'Maori Religion and Mythology', London: Longmans, Green and Co. 1882
[49] T. W. Thompson, Journal of the Gypsy Folklore Society VIII (1929), pp. 33-39.
[50] Caesar, Bellum Gallicum VI. 18 quoted by Eli Edward Burriss, 'Taboo, Magic, Spirits: A Study of Primitive Elements in Roman Religion'
[51] Satyricon LXIII. & Lucan, Bellum Civile VI. 557-558 quoted by Eli Edward Burriss
[52] Fasti VI. 155-162. quoted by Eli Edward Burriss
[53] St Augustine, 'De Civitate Dei VI. 9.' quoted by Eli Edward Burriss
[54] Walter Gregor, 'Notes on the Folklore of the Northeast of Scotland', London: Folklore Society, 1881
[55] John Valentine Merbitz, 'De Infantibus Supposititiis, vulgo Wechsel~Bälgen,' Dresden, 1678, quoted by Charles Godfrey Leland in 'Gypsy Lore…'
[56] Thomas Johnson Westropp, 'A Study of Folklore on the Coasts of Connacht, Ireland' Folklore: A Quarterly Review, vol. 32, 1921
[57] J. F. Campbell, 'Popular Tales of the West Highlands', as published in George Douglas, 'Scottish Fairy and Folk Tales' London, Walter Scott Publishing Co., 1901
[58] Sir Walter Scott, 'On the Fairies of Popular Superstition' Edinburgh: Ballantyne, 1833, vol. 2
[59] James MacDougall, 'Folk Tales and Fairy Lore in Gaelic and English', Edinburgh: John Grant, 1910
[60] William Henderson, 'Notes of the Folklore of the Northern Counties of England and the Borders' London: Folklore Society, 1879
[61] Many thanks to Michael at www.astrology-numerology.com for his assistance
[62] Jean Briggs, 'Living Dangerously: The Introductory Foundations of Value in Canadian Intuit Society.' In Eleanor Leacock and Richard Lee, Eds., Politics and History in Band Societies. New York: Columbia University Press, 1982, p. 117.
[63] John Jones, 'Medical, Philosophical and Vulgar Errors of Various Kinds' London,: 1797
[64] Jamieson Scottish Dictionary, iii. 300.
[65] W. J. Hoffman, M. D. 'Folk-lore of the Pennsylvania Germans' Part I: Journal of American Folklore 1:2 pp. 125-35 [1888] Part II: Journal of American Folklore 2:4 pp. 23-35 [1889]
[66] County Folklore, vol. 3: Examples of Printed Folklore Concerning the Orkney & Shetland Islands, collected by G. F. Black and edited by Northcote W. Thomas, London: Folklore Society, 1903

Printed in the United Kingdom
by Lightning Source UK Ltd.
104090UKS00001B/385-408